Medical Kirundi

Phrasebook and Glossary

first edition 2014

ISBN is 1500731587
EAN-13 is 978-1500731588

by A.H.Zemback

Thanks to Dr. Blaise Machel Bisabwa for his assistance.

Introduction/ demographics	English	Kirundi
	How are you?	N'amaki? (N'amahoro?)
	Good morning, good afternoon	Bgakeye, mwiriwe,
	My name is ...	Nitwa...
	I am a... (1)nurse, (2)doctor, (3)social worker, (4)dentist, (5)eye doctor, (6)surgeon, (7) physical therapist	Ndi...1) umuforomo 2) umuganga 3) umufasha w'abantu mu ngorane zinyranye 4) umuganga w'amenyo 5) umuganga w'amaso 6) umuganga ubaga 7)muganga gorora abamugaye
	What is your name?	Witwa nde?
	Can you write your name in English?	Urashobora kwandika izina ryawe mu congereya?
	I am pleased to meet you.	Ndaryohewe nuko duhuye.
	Please write your name here.	Mwandike izina ryanyu hano
	Do you speak English?	Muravuga icongereza?
	I don't speak Kirundi.	Ntakirundi mvuga?
	Say that one more time, please.	Mwoshobora gusubiramwo rimwe?
	I don't understand.	Sinumva.
	Can you speak slowly, please?	Vuga buke buke ndabasavye.
	Come with me.	Ingo tujane.
	Sit down, please.	Ni mwicare.
	What province do you live in?	Muba muyihe ntara?
	What is your address?	Uba hehe? (Vuga aho uba.)
	Who else lives at your home?	Nibande mubana i wanyu?
	What is your telephone number? (Say your number.)	Telephone yawe ni iyihe? (Tanga telephone yawe.)
	Do you have an I.D?	Murafise ibibaranga?
	Can you give us the name and telephone number or address of someone to be contacted?	Mwoshobora kuduha izina na numero ya terefone canke muturangire uwo twokwitura?
	Are you married?	Murubatse?
	What is your age?	Ufise imyaka ingahe?

Chief complaint	English	Kirundi
	chief complaint	ingorane nyamukuru
	What is your emergency?	Ufise ingorane ki?
	What is your health concern today?	Waje gukora iki uyu musi?
	When did this problem start?	Iyo ngorane yatanguye ryari?
	How many days have you been feeling ill?	Haheze imisi ingahe wumva kurwaye?
	Have you had an accident?	Woba waragize isanganya?
	Is this injury from a landmine?	Iki gikomere catewe n igisasu bateze?
	Were you shot with a gun?	Barakurashe?
	Is this from a machete?	Baragutemye n umupanga?
	Is this from a car accident?	Vyavuye kw isanganya ry umuduga
	Did you lose consciousness after this happened?	Woba warataye ubwenge bimaze kuba?
	Did you lose a lot of blood before coming here?	Woba waratakaje amaraso menshi imbere yokuza ngaha?
	What medicine have you taken?	Wafashe uwuhe muti?
	Do you have any pain?	Hari ububabare ufise?
	When did the pain start (use the calendar to show me)?	Ububabare bwatanguye ryar(koresha ikiranga misi mukunyereka)?
	How many days have you had the pain?	Wamaranye ububabare imisi ingana gute?
	What is your level of pain? 0= no pain, 10 = severe pain	Wumva urugero rw ububabare bwawe rungana gute?0=ntabubabare, 10=wumva ububabare burengenje.
	Hold up the number of fingers.	Fata igitigiri c intoke.
	Is the pain severe?	Ububabare ni bwinshi?
	Is your pain burning?	Wumva ububabare bumeze nkubushe?
	Is the pain constant...?	Ububabare bugumaho?
	or does it come and go?	iraza kandi ikagenda?
	Does the pain go to your back?	Ububabare buraja no mu mugongo?
	Touch the spot where it hurts with one finger.	Korako n urutoke aho ubabara cane.
	What makes it better?	N 'iki kibugabanya?
	What makes it worse?	N 'iki kivyunyura,kigusonga?
	When do you get the pain...	Ubabara ryari.....
	at night, before meals, after meals?	mw ijoro,imbere yo gufungura,uhejeje gufungura?

5

Chief complaint	English	Kirundi
	Have you seen a doctor for this problem before?	Wabonye uwundi muganga w'iyo ngorane?
	Have you taken medicine for this problem before?	Wafashe umuti w'iyo ngorane?
	Have you been in the hospital before?	Wagumye mu bitaro imbere?
	What were you treated for?	Bakuvuye iki?
	Is anyone else sick at home?	Nta wundi agwaye i wawe?

Common complaints	English	Kirundi
	My lower back hurts.	Ndababara mu kiyunguyungu.
	My neck is stiff.	Izosi ryanje riradadaraye.
	I have a fever	Ndashushe.
	I have night sweats.	Ndabira intungumba mwijoro.
	It hurts when I swallow.	Ndababara ndiko ndamira.
	I have an earache.	Ndababara mu gutwi.
	I have poor vision.	Simbona neza.
	I have a toothache.	Iryinyo rirandya.
	My tooth is loose.	Hari iryinyo mbura.
	My dentures are loose and my gums hurt.	Amenyo yanje yarahongotse kandi n ikinyigishi kirambabaza.
	My gums bleed when I brush my teeth.	Ikinyigishi canje kirava amaraso iyo ndiko ndiyugumura.
	I have shoulder pain.	Ndababara kurutugu.
	I have elbow pain.	Ndababara mu nkokora
	I have wrist pain	Ndababara kugikonjo
	I have knee pain.	Ndababara mw ivi
	I have ankle pain.	Ndababara kujisho ryikirenge
	I am dizzy.	Ndazungurirwa
	I am very nervous.	Numvishavu ryinshi
	I can't sleep.	Sinshobora gusinzira
	I am tired.	Ndarushe
	I have chest pain.	Ndababara mu gakiriza
	My heart beats very fast.	Umutima wanje uriruka cane.
	I have a headache.	Ndamenetse umutwe.
	I have trouble breathing.	Mpema nabi.
	I am short of breath at night.	Birangora guhema mwijoro.
	I am short of breath with exertion.	Birangora guhema nkoze ikintu kiruhisha.
	I have to sleep sitting up.	Ntegerezwa gusinzira nicaye.
	I am coughing a lot.	Ndakorora cane.
	It hurts when I cough.	Ndababara iyo nkoroye.
	I have not had a menstrual cycle for ... months.	Haheze...... amezi ntabona amaraso or ntaja mubutinyanka.
	I think I am pregnant.	Nibaza ko nibungenze.
	I have morning sickness.	Mvyuka ndwaye.
	I am pregnant	Ndibungenze.
	I have pain during my menstrual period.	Ndababara iyo ndi mubutinyanka or ndababara iyo ndi mu maraso.

7

Common complaints	English	Kirundi
	I have a vaginal infection.	Ndarwaye mu gihimba c irondoka.
	I am on a birth control pill.	Ndiko ndafata ibinini vyo kuvyara kurugero.
	I have a stomach ache (cramp).	mu'nda harahotera
	I cannot eat.	Ntibikunda ko mfungura
	I have heartburn.	Ndasha kumutima
	I am nauseated.	Mfise iseseme
	I have been vomiting.	Namye ndadahwa
	I have been vomiting worms.	Namye ndadahwa inzoka
	I have indigestion.	Numva nuzuye inda
	I have no appetite.	Ntakayabagu mfise
	I have diarrhea.	Ndacibwamwo
	I am suffering from constipation.	Ndagumiwe
	I have blood in my stool.	Harimwo amaraso mu musarani wanje
	My stools are light colored.	umwanda mukuru harimwo amabara
	I get up at night to urinate.	Ndavyuka kwihagarika mwijoro
	My urine is cloudy.	umukoyo wanje usa nabi
	I have bloody urine.	Umukoyo wanje urimwo amaraso
	I have pain with urination.	Ndababara kumwanda muto or Ndabababa ndiko ndihagarika
	I feel sick.	Numva ndwaye
	I feel weak.	Numva atantenge mfise
	I have pain here.	Ndababara ngaha
	I think I broke my arm.	Ndakeka konavunye ukuboko kwanje
	I think I broke my leg.	Ndakeka konavunye ukuguru kwanje
	I have a rash.	Mfise uruherehere
	I have a burn.	Mfise ubushe
	I have a wound.	Mfise igikomere
	I am injured.	Nakomeretse
	He hurt his head.	Yisetse
	He is unconscious.	Yataye ubwenge
	He is bleeding a lot.	Ariko arava amaraso
	He has a broken bone.	Afise igufa ryavunitse
	My baby nurses well.	Umwana wanje yonka neza
	My baby suckles poorly.	Umwana wanje yonka nabi
	I don't have enough (breast) milk.	Ntamaberebere akwiye mfise
	I need a breast pump so I can get milk for the baby.	Nkeneye ico nokamisha kugira ndonke amaberebere y umwana.

Past Medical and Surgical History	English	Kirundi
	Do you have any chronic health problems?	Ufise indwara umwanya muremure?
	Do you have a history of:	Warigeze urwara
	AIDS	SIDA
	anemia	indwara yo gukama amaraso
	angina	ibimiromiro
	arthritis	indwara ifata amahuriro y'amagufwa
	asthma	asima
	bronchitis	indwara yo mu mahaha
	cancer	kansere
	chicken pox	agasama
	cholera	korera
	common cold; viral uri	agahehera
	congestive heart failure	uguhagarara umutima
	depression	akabonge
	diabetes mellitus	indwara y'igisukari
	diphtheria	diptheria (ikirato)
	eczema	izabana
	epilepsy	intandara
	gonorrhea	agaswende; mburugu
	heart murmur	ikiriro
	heart problems	indwara y'umutima
	hepatitis	indwara y'igitigu
	herpes simplex	umugera wa herpes
	hypertension	umutima uratera vuba
	insect bite	gukomorwa n agakoko
	jaundice	umuhondo
	malaria	inyonko
	measles	agasama
	mumps	amasambambwika
	paratyphoid fever	indwara yisuku rike
	peritonsillar abscess	igihute co mumagage
	pneumonia	umusonga
	polio	ubukangwe
	rabies	indwara iterwa no kurumwa n'inyamaswa
	ringworm	inzoka zo munda
	scabies (also used for skin rash)	mbandakara
	scarlet fever	indwara y ubushihe

Past Medical and Surgical History	English	Kirundi
	stroke	n'indwara bukumbi y'ubwonko
	syphilis	agashangara; isofisi
	tapeworm	inzoka; igikangaga
	thyroid disease	umwingo
	tonsillitis	indwara yo mu magage
	tuberculosis	igituntu
	typhoid fever	sutama
	warts	isununu
	whooping cough (pertussis)	inkorora y'akanira
	worms (roundworm)	inzoka
	yellow fever	indwara y ubushihe
	Do you know what HIV means?	Woba uzi ico HIV gisigura?
	Have you been tested for HIV?	Waripimishije umugera wa SIDA?
	Are you infected with HIV ?	Woba waranduye umugera wa SIDA?
	You need a blood test to check for HIV.	Urakeneye igipimo c amaraso kugira wipimishe SIDA
	HIV/AIDS	Umugera wa Sida
	Date starting ARV?	Watanguye ryari imiti y umugera (ARV)?
	Date and value of last CD4?	Itariki nurugero vyanyuma vya CD4?
	Do you have a vaccination record?	Woba ufise urupapuro rw incandarwa?
	Have you have pneumonia or meningitis?	Woba waragwaye umusonga canke mugiga?
	Have you had surgery in the past?	Warigeze kubagwa?
	What surgery was done?	Bagukoze iki? or Bakubaze iki?

Family/social history	English	Kirundi
	Is your mother living?	Uracafise nyoko?
	Is your father living?	Uracafise so?
	What did your father/mother die from?	So\ Nyoko yishwe n iki?
	Do your brothers/sisters have health problems?	Basazawe\Bashikawe boba bagwaye?
	Do you have any children?	Urafise abana?
	What is your religion?	Usengera he?
	Do you drink alcohol?	Uranywa inzoga?
	How many drinks per day?	Zingahe kumusi?
	Do you drink alcohol every day?	Woba unywa inzoga buri musi?
	Do you smoke cigarettes?	Uranywa itabi?
	How many cigarettes per day?	Zingahe ku musi?
	What kind of work do you do?	Ukora iki?

Medications/ allergies	English	Kirundi
	I am allergic to...	Simbonana na.......ncandwara.
	Have you had reactions to medications?	Uramaze gufata imiti hanyuma ikakugirira ingaruka mbi?
	What is the name of the medication that you had the reaction to?	Ni uwuhe muti wakumereye nabi?
	Are you allergic to any medicine?	Hari umuti ukumerera nabi?
	Do you take any medication every day?	Urafata umuti imisi yose?
	Do you take (modern) medication at home?	Hari umuti(w ikizungu) uriko urafatira muhira?
	Which medication?	Uwuhe muti?
	Have you taken traditional medication?	Hari umuti w ikirundi wigeze ufata?
	Are you taking Bactrim?	Hari Bactrim uriko urafata?
	I want to see the medication bottle.	Nshaka kuraba agacupa kuwo muti

Review of systems: lymph, bone, blood	English	Kirundi
	Do you have skin problems?	Hari indwara zo kurukoba ufise?
	Do you have a rash?	Hari uruherehere ufise?
	Do you have any blisters or sores?	Har imisonga wumva?
	Do you have any problems with dry skin?	Hari ingorane yo kwuma urukoba wigera ugira?
	Do you have itching?	Uraribwa ku mubiri?
	Have you been bitten by ticks?	Uramaze kuribwa n inyondwi?
	Have you seen any rats in your home?	Hari imbeba urigera ubona mu nzu iwawe?
	Were you bitten by a dog or another animal?	Uramaze kuribwa n imbwa canke ikindi gikoko?
	Do you have lymph node enlargement or pain?	Hari amasumbi ufise canke ububabare?
	Do you have bone pain?	Urababara igufa?
	Do you have joint pain?	Uraribwa mu ngingo?
	Do you have joint swelling?	Uravyimvye mu ngingo?
	Do you have muscle pain?	Urababara umutsi?
	Where is the muscle pain?	Ububabare bw umutsi butumbereye he?
	Do you have pain in the back or the neck?	Hari ububabare ufise mu mugongo canke kw izosi?
	Have you ever had a blood transfusion?	Warigeze uterwa amaraso?
	Do you have bleeding problems?	Hari ingorane yo kuva amaraso ufise?
	Do you have a problem with bleeding easily?	Urava amaraso cane muri rusangi?
	Do you have bleeding from anywhere?	Hari amaraso aca irya n ino ufise?
	Do you urinate frequently?	Uja kwihagarika kenshi?
	Are you very thirsty?	Uranyoterwa cane?
	Have you lost weight?	Warataye ibiro?
	Is the ankle pain so severe you cannot walk on it?	Ububabare bwo kujisho ry ikirenge wumva bukubuza gutambuka?
	Does your knee give way?	Warigeze kugira inda?
	Do you feel pain when you move your shoulder?	Urababara uhindukije igitugu?
	Have you had any broken bones?	Warigeze uvunika amagufa?
	What bones were broken?	Ni ayahe magufa yavunitse?

Review of systems: HEENT	English	Kirundi
	Have you suffered from a head trauma in the past?	Warigeze ugira isanga ukababara umutwe muri kahise?
	Do you have dizziness?	Urafise ibizunguzungu?
	Have you blacked-out?	Uraraba ubwenge?
	Do you have vision problems?	Hari ingorane zo kubona ufise?
	Is your vision good in both eyes?	Urabona neza ku maso yose?
	Which eye is problematic?	Ni irihe jisho rifise ikibazo?
	Do you have vision loss?	Woba ufise ingorane yo kutabona neza?
	Do you have double vision?	Hari ubwo ubonamwo ikintu bibiri?
	Do you have pain in bright light?	Uragira ikibazo c umuco mwinshi?
	Do you have spots in front of your eyes?	Hari inzatsa ubona imbere yawe?
	Do you have blurred vision?	Ubona ivyijiji?
	Do your eyes water a lot?	Uragira amosozi menshi?
	Do you have pain in your eyes?	Urababara mu maso?
	Do you wear glasses?	Urambara amarori?
	Do you use contact lenses?	Hari rantiye ukoresha?
	Can you hear well?	Urumva neza?
	Do you have hearing problems?	Hari ingorane zo kwumva ufise?
	Which ear is effected?	Ni ukuhe gutwi kugwaye?
	Do you have pain in your ears?	Urababara mu matwi?
	Do you have drainage from your ears?	Hari ibiseseka biva mu gutwi?
	Do you have hearing loss in only one ear?	Ufise ugutwi kumwe kwonyene kutumva?
	Do you have buzzing in the ears?	Hari iminzerere wumva mu matwi?
	Do you have a runny nose?	Uragira ibicurane?
	Do you have nosebleeds?	Hari umwuna ufise?
	Do you have bleeding gums?	Ufise ibinyigishi biva amaraso?
	Do you have ulcers in your mouth?	Hari ibisebe ufise mu kanwa?
	Do you have a toothache?	Urababara iryinyo?
	Do you have a broken tooth?	Urafise iryinyo ryacitse?
	Do you have lumps or swelling in your mouth?	Hari imisonga canke ikivyimba ufise mu kanwa?
	Do you have hoarseness (a change in your voice)?	Urasarara?
	Do you have a sore throat?	Urababara mumihogo?
	Do you have neck stiffness?	Uradadarara kw izosi?

Review of systems: respiratory/cardiac	English	Kirundi
	Are you short of breath?	Urahema nabi?
	Do you have difficulty breathing when you lay down?	Urahema nabi iyo uryamye?
	Do you have pain when you take a deep breath?	Urababara uhemye cane?
	Do you have wheezing?	Urahezera?
	Do you have a cough?	Urakorora?
	How long have you had the cough?	Umaranye igihe kingana gute inkorora?
	Do you cough up phlegm?	Urakorora?
	Do you have a lot of sputum?	Ufise ibikororwa vyinshi?
	Do you have bloody sputum?	Igikororwa kirimwo amaraso?
	What color is your sputum.	Igikororwa cawe gisa gute?
	Have you had tuberculosis?	Wari ufise igituntu?
	Where did you receive treatment?	Waronkeye imiti he?
	How many months did you take the medication?	Wabifashe amezi angahe?
	Do you have chest pain?	Ubabara igikiriza?
	Do you have pain that radiates from your chest to your left arm?	Hari ububabare buva mu gikiriza bushwara ukuboko kw ukubamfu ufise?
	Do you sweat when you have this chest pain?	Urabira icuya igihe ufise ubwo bubabare?
	Do you have palpitations?	Umutima wawe uradidagizwa cane?
	Do you have leg edema?	Uravyimvye amaguru?
	Do you have weakness?	Uracika imitsi?
	Do you have fatigue?	Ufise uburuhe?

Review of systems: GI/GU	English	Kirundi
	Are you eating well?	Urafungura neza?
	Are you drinking well?	Uranywa neza?
	Do you have abdominal pain?	Urababara mu unda? Urababara umushishito?
	Do you have abdominal pain after you eat?	Urababara umushishito agiheza gufungura?
	When did this problem start?	Iyo ngorane yatanguye ryari?
	Has it been weeks, months, years?	Bimaze indwi,amezi,imyaka?
	Are you in pain now?	Urumva ububabare ubu?
	Touch the spot where you have pain with one finger.	Korako n urutoke aho wumva ubabara.
	Does it hurt all the time?	Ubabara umwanya wose?
	Does the pain come and go?	Ububabare burahera bukagaruka?
	Is the pain better than yesterday?	Wumva ububabare bwagabanutse ugereranije n ejo?
	Do you have fever?	Urashuha?
	How many days have you had a fever?	Umaranye umucanwa iminsi ingahe?
	Do you have chills?	Urajugumira? Urahinda umushitsi?
	Do you have night sweats?	Uradugumbigwa mw'ijoro?
	Have you lost your appetite?	Urabura akayabagu?
	Have you vomited?	Urayogwa?
	Is your vomit bloody or black?	Udahwa amaraso canke ivyirabura?
	Have you vomited blood?	Wadashwe amaraso?
	Do you have nausea?	Ufise iseseme? Urasesemwa?
	Did the nausea start today?	Iseseme ryatanguye uyu munsi?
	How many days have you been nauseated?	Umaze iminsi ingahe usesemwa?
	Do you have bloating?	Uruzura inda?
	Did you have a bowel movement today?	Wahemye uyu munsi? Or Wasuze uyu munsi?
	When was your last stool?	Uheruka kwituma ubwanyuma ryari?
	Are you constipated?	Uragumiwe?
	Can you pass gas?	Urashobora guhema? Or Urashobora gusura?
	Do you have diarrhea?	Uracibwamwo?
	How many times per day?	Kangahe kumunsi?
	Have you passed any black stools?	Wigeze ugira umwanda mukuru wirabura?
	Are your stools bloody?	Ufise amaraso mu mazirantoke?

Review of systems: GI/GU	English	Kirundi
	What color is your stool...1) red 2) yellow 3) green 4) black?	Umwanda mukuru / umusarani wawe usa gute....1)uratukura 2)usa numuhondo 3)usa nicatsi kibisi 4)urirabura?
	Do you have anal itching?	Uriyaga mu gisusu?
	Do you have pain with swallowing?	Urababara uriko uramira?
	Do you have difficulty swallowing?	Hari ingorane ufise mukumira?
	Do you have a burning pain in your stomach?	Hari ubushe wumva mu mushishito?
	Are you hungry?	Urashonje?
	When did you last eat?	Uheruka gufungura ryari?
	Have you seen worms in your stools? (Do you have worms?)	Hari inzoka wabonye mu musarani wawe?(Hari inzoka ufise?)
	Have you had a gastroscopy?	Barigeze bakumurika mu nda?
	Are you urinating well?	Urihagarika neza?
	Do you have pain when you urinate?	Urababara iyo uriko urihagarika?
	Do you have a burning sensation when you urinate?	Hari ubushe wumva uriko urihagarika/ urasoba?
	Do you have a sore on your penis?	Urababara ku nzanyi?
	Do you have dark urine?	Umukoyo wawe urirabura?
	What does your urine look like?	Umukoyo wawe usa gute?
	Is your urine cloudy?	Umukoyo wawe usa nabi?
	Do you have sharp pains in your back where the last rib meets the spine?	Hari ububabare ufise mu mugongo aho urubavu rwanyuma ruhurira n uruti rw umugongo?
	Does the pain go to your scrotum?	Ububabare bushwara mw ivya?
	Do you have difficulty starting to urinate?	Uragira ingorane yo gutangura gusoba?
	Do you have dribbling after you finish?	Urababwa uhejeje ?
	How often do you urinate at night?	Usoba/wihagarika kangahe mwijoro?
	Do you have the urge to urinate but can't pass any urine?	Urumva ko ushaka gusoba/kwihagarika vyihuta mugabo bikanka ko haza n akama?
	Is the urine stream slow?	Umukoyo rsohoka bukebuke?
	Have you urinated today?	Wihagaritse/wasovye uyu munsi?
	Does your bladder feel full?	Wumva agasaho kumukoyo kuzuye?
	Do you leak urine when you cough or sneeze?	Hari ubwo umukoyo ugutanga iyo ukoroye canke wasamuye?
	Do you have blood in the urine?	Urava amaraso iyo uriko urihagarika?
	Have you every passed a kidney stone?	Uramaze gusohoka akabuye kumukoyo?
	Do you have incontinence?	Urisobako

Review of systems:Women's Health	English	Kirundi
	Have you noticed any breast lumps?	Uramaze kwumva utuvyimba mu ma bere?
	Do you have nipple discharge?	Hari ibizibizi biva mumabere?
	Do you have swelling around or below your nipples?	Ntatuvyimva wumva mumabere?
	Have you reached change of life?	Warashoboye guhindura ubuzima?
	Are you having vaginal bleeding?	Hari amaraso ava mu gitereko?
	How long have you had the bleeding?	Kuva ryari uva amaraso mu gitereko?
	Is the vaginal bleeding continuous or does it come and go?	Ayo maraso aguma aza canke aragenda hama akagaruka?
	Have you missed your menstrual period recently?	Uramaze gusiba ukwezi utagiye mu maraso?
	Are you pregnant?	Uribungenze?
	How many months pregnant are you?	Mufise imbanyi y amezi angahe?
	Could you possibly be pregnant?	Murashobora kwibungenga?
	Can we do a pregnancy test?	Turashobora gugupima ko wibungenze?
	Are your periods regular?	Ubuna amaraso buri kwezi kumatariki asa?
	Are your periods painful?	Urababara uri mukwezi?
	Is the flow heavy?	Haza menshi cane?
	When did your last period start?	Uheruka amaraso yanyuma ryari?
	How many days do your periods last?	Umara imnsi ingahe mumaraso?
	Do you bleed between periods?	Urava amaraso hagati mukwezi?
	Do you take birth control pills?	Hari ibinini vzo kurinda kuvyara intahekana ufata?
	Do you have an intrauterine device (IUD)?	Hari agashinge bagushizemwo?
	Do you have pain during intercourse?	Urababara muriko murarangura amabanga yabubatse?
	Do you have vaginal itching?	Uriyagaza mubihimba vyirondoka

18

Review of systems: Women's Health	English	Kirundi
	Do you have vaginal pain?	Urababara mubihimba vyirondoka?
	Do you have unusual discharge from the vagina; a little or a lot?	Hari ibizi biva mugihimba cirondoka? Bingana gute?
	How many times have you been pregnant?	Imbanyi mwibungenze ifise amezi angahe?
	How many children do you have?	Mufise abana bangahe?
	Were your deliveries normal?	Abana bose mwabavyaye neza?
	Have you had any miscarriages?	Hamaze kuvayo zingahe?
	Did you have problems in your previous pregnancies?	Haringorane wagize kumbayi za kera?
	Did you have any severe bleeding after any of your deliveries?	Hari amaraso menshi wigeze uva uhejeje kwibaruka?
	Do you know your blood type?	Urazi umurwi wamaraso yawe?
	Do you have ankle swelling?	Uravyimba amaguru?
	Are you in labor?	Uri ku gise?
	When did your contractions start?	Ibise vyatnanguye ryari?
	Are the contractions regular or irregular?	Ibise biya buri mwanya canke birateba?
	Did your water break?	Kumena agasho k'amazi?
	Is this your first baby?	Uyu mwana nuwambere?
	Do you feel the baby move?	Urumva umwana akina munda?
	Do not push.	Ntutere?
	Push now.	Tera ubu.
	Push very hard.	Tera cane.
	You have a boy!	Wavyaye umuungu!
	You have a girl!	Wavyaye umukobwa!
	You have twins!	Wavyaye amahasa!
	The baby/babies is/are healthy.	Abana bawe bameze neza.

Review of systems: neonatal and peripartum	English	Kirundi
	How old is your baby?	Umwana wawe afise imyaka ingahe?
	Was your baby born at home or the health center?	Umwana wawe yavukiye muhira canke kwa muganga?
	What was your baby's birth weight?	Umwana yavukanye ibiro bingahe?
	How are you feeding the baby, with breast or bottle?	Umwana umwonsa gute? Umuha ibere canke mw ibibero?
	Is the baby nursing well?	Umwana aronka neza?
	Has the baby had a convulsion?	Umwana aramaze gufatwa nibisahuzi?
	What color was the amniotic fluid?	Amazi yumwana yasa gute?
	Were you ill before the delivery?	Wararwaye imbere yo kwibaruka?
	What is the baby's temperature.	Umwana yavukanye ubushuhe bungana gute?
	Your baby is sick.	Umwana wawe ararwaye
	We need to help your baby.	Dushaka kuvura umwana wawe
	You can stay with the baby.	Urashobora gusigarana numwana wawe.
	We need to warm the baby up.	Dushaka gushuhisha umwana wawe.
	We need to put the baby under a special light to because the skin color is yellow.	Dushaka gushira umwana munsi yitara, kubera urukoba rwiwe rusa numuhondo.
	We need to give the baby oxygen.	Dushaka guha umwana wawe umwuka.
	Does the child cry often?	Umwana arakunda kurira?
	Is the child gaining weight?	Umwana arunguka ibiro?
	Does the child have a good appetite?	Umwana arafise akayabagu?
	Did the child eat today...yesterday?	Umwana yafunguye ?
	What kinds of pain does the child complain of?	Umwana ababara hehe?
	Is the child drinking ok?	Umwana ababara hehe?
	Is the child eating ok?	Umwana arafungura neza?
	Have you seen worms in the vomit or stool? (Does he have worms?)	Uramaze kubona inzoka mu bidahwe canke mu mwanda mukuru?
	Did your child pass urine today?	Umwana yasonvye uyu munsi?

Review of systems: neonatal and peripartum	English	Kirundi
	Did you child have a stool today/yesterday?	Umwana wawe yasohotse uyu munsi?
	Does he/she have diarrhea?	Uracibwamo?
	Has he/she been vomiting?	Uradahwa?
	Do you have the baby's vaccine card?	Urafie impapuro umwana yacandagiweko?

Review of systems: neuro & psychiatric	English	Kirundi
	Do you have facial weakness?	Urajonjogoye?
	Do you have facial numbness?	Wumva mu maso hakeye?
	Do you have leg weakness?	Wumva ufise inguvu mu maguru?
	Do you have leg numbness?	Uravyumva ku maguru yawe mu bisanzwe? Wumva utadegedwa mumaguru?
	Do you have arm weakness?	Wummva ufise inguvu mu kuboko?
	Do you have arm numbness?	Wumva mumaboko hadakongataye?
	Did you lose consciousness?	Urata ubwenge?
	Have you had any convulsions?	Uramaze gufatwa n ibisahuzi?
	Do you have tremors?	Uratetemera?
	Do you have headaches?	Urameneka umutwe?
	Have you had vision loss in one eye?	Hari ijisho ryoba ritabone neza?
	Do you have problems with your balance?	Haringorane ufise no gutambuka?
	Do you feel dizzy?	Urazungurirwa?
	Do you have problems walking?	Urafise ingorane zo gutambuka?
	Do you have pain that travels from your buttock down the back of your leg?	Hari ububabare buva inyuma kugisusu bumanuka kukuguru?
	Do you have memory problems?	Hari ingorane yo kwibagira ufise?
	Do you have anxiety?	Wumva utatekanye?
	Do you have depression?	Wumva wayinze?
	How is your mood?	Wumva umeze gute?
	Do you hear voices (that others don't hear)?	Hari amajwi wumva abandi batariko barayumva?
	Do you sleep well?	Urasinzira neza?

English	Kirundi
Lay down.	Ryama ugaramye.
Sit up (if they are laying down).	Vyuka wicare.
Stand up.	Hagarara. (Haguruka)
Sit down.	Icara.
Sit here.	Icara aha.
Open your mouth.	Asama.
Show your tongue.	Nyereka ururimi.
Say "ahh".	Vuga uti "ahh".
Breathe deeply.	Hezuka cane.
Close your eyes.	Humiriza.
Raise your eyebrows.	Duza inkokora.
Smile widely.	Twenga cane.
Swallow now.	Mira ubu naho.
Open your eyes.	Kanura.
Say "yes" if you feel this.	Vuga "ego" niwumva iki.
Do this movement (quickly).	Gira gutya.
Move your arm like I do.	Hindukiza ukuboko nkuko ngize.
Lay on your side.	Ryamira urubavu.
Lay on your abdomen.	Ryama wubitse inda.
Bend your knee.	Pfunya ivi.

Physical exam	English	Kirundi
General	Appearance, height	isura, uburebure
Weight	weight (pounds/kilograms) "Stand on the scale."	Ibiro"Hagarara ku munzane"
Vital signs	pulse, blood pressure "I need to check your blood pressure" respiratory rate	Urugero umutima utererako, umurindi wamaraso. Ngira ndagufatire umurindi wamaraso
Vital signs	temperature "Hold this under your tongue."	ubushuhe bwumubiri
Skin	skin	umubiri
HEENT	visual acuity "Cover your right eye. Read this. Now, cover your left eye." (Show them a Snellen chart)	Igice cukuboneramwo. "Fuka ijisho ry iburyo. Soma ibi. Ubu naho, fuka ijisho ry ibubamfu"
HEENT	conjunctivae, sclerae	igice cera c ijisho
HEENT	pupils	imbonero
HEENT	PERRL pupils equal, round and reactive to light	ingene imbonero zifata zegereze umuco
HEENT	"I am going to put some drops in your eyes."	"Ngire ndagushirire umutı mu maso."
HEENT	"You are going to feel a puff of air in your eyes."	"Uraza kwumva impemu nyinshi mumaso yawe."
HEENT	optic disc (exam using an ophthalmoscope)	igipimo c amaso
HEENT	ear canal, tympanic membrane	iyomviro
HEENT	AC> BC bilaterally? Rinne. "Cover this ear with your hand. Tell me when you cannot feel the vibration." Move the tuning fork off the mastoid process and next to but not touching the ear. "Tell me when the sound stops."	Ugara uku gutwi nukuboko kwawe. Urambarira udashoboye kwumva igitetemera.
HEENT	Weber "Is the sound the same in both ears?	"Wumva neza, cokimwe mu matwi yose."
HEENT	nasal mucosa (inside of the nose) "I am going to look into your nose."	Inyama yo mumazuru. "Ngira ndabe muzuru ryawe."
HEENT	nasal septum	inyama igabura amazuru
HEENT	soft palate	igice co muzuru
HEENT	sinuses (cavity behind the forehead)	ibihima ubwonko buhemeramwo

Physical exam	English	Kirundi
HEENT	teeth	amenyo
HEENT	1) mouth or lips, 2) gums, 3) teeth, 4)uvula, Stenson's and Wharton's ducts "Open your mouth, please."	1. umunwa 2.ibishinyi. 3. amenyo. 4. akamirampeke, uturingoti dusuka amate mukanwa. "Ndagusavye wasame."
HEENT	"Stick out your tongue please."	"Asama usohore ururimi."
HEENT	"Say ahh!"	"Vuga ahh!"
Chest	Auscultation,(listen to the lungs) "Breathe in deeply."	Gupima amahaha. "Hema cane."
Chest	percussion "I must tap on your chest- this won't hurt."	Kudodora umubiri:"Gupima ibihimba vyimbere mugikiriza no munda."
Chest	"Lie down on your back, please."	"Ryama ugaramye, ndakwinginze." (Woshobora kuryama ugaramye.)
Chest	"Lie on your left side."	"Ryamira urubavu rw ukubamfu."
Chest	"Lie on your right side."	"Ryamira urubavu rw iburyo."
Chest	"Does it hurt here?"	"Ni ng'aha ubabara?" ("Urababara ngaha?")
Chest	cva tenderness (where the last rib meets the spine)	Aho akagufa kanyuma kigikiriza gahurira n uruti rwumugongo.
Chest	heart rate, rhythm "I need to listen to your chest. Breathe normally."	urugero umutima utererako
Chest	heart murmur?	ikiriro?
Chest	carotid "Hold your breath."	"Pfunga impwemu."
Chest	jugular venous pressure (pressure in the neck vein)	inguvu zumurindi wamaraso ava mubwonko
Chest	nipple discharge?	Hari ivyisesa biva mw imoko?
Chest	breast tenderness?	kuvyimba amabere
Chest	breast exam	gupima amabere
Vascular	carotid, radial, aortic pulsation "Hold your breath."	ibice umurindi wamaraso utereramwo: kwizosi, kukuboko, mu gikiriya. "Hagarika guhema"
Vascular	femoral, dorsalis pedis and posterior tibial pulsation (pulsation of legs)	ibice umurindi wamaraso utereramwo kukuguru? Kwitako, ku kirenge, kumurundi
Extremities	leg edema?	Kuvyimba amaguru
Extremities	"Lie down please."	"Ryama ugaramye, ndakwinginze." (Woshobora kuryama ugaramye.)
Pain	"Show me where it hurts, by touching the spot with one finger."	"Nyereka aho ubabara, mukuhakora nurutoke."
Pain	"Does this hurt?"	"Urababara ngaha?"
Abdomen	umbilicus	umukondo
Abdomen	inguinal hernia?	Umusipa

25

Physical exam	English	Kirundi
Abdomen	palpation "I must press my hands on your abdomen."	gukanda. "Ntegereza gukanda munda yawe nintoke"
Abdomen	auscultation "I must listen to your abdomen."	kwumviriza munda. "Ntegerezwa kwumviriza munda zawe."
Abdomen	fluid wave, superficial abdominal veins?	umukuba wamazi yo munda, imitzs yo kunda hejuru
Women's health	Uterine height (cm)	uburebure bw imbanyi
Women's health	fetal heart tones	uguhema kw umwana
Women's health	presentation:	ingene umwana yicaye
Women's health	face presentation	gutanguza amaso
Women's health	breech presentation	umwana yicaye
Women's health	speculum exam	ugupima igikororwa
Women's health	vaginal exam	ugupima mu gihimba cirondoka
Women's health	gestational age	ameyi imbanyi ifise
Women's health	amniotic fluid (waters within)	uruziruzi
Neonatal	Apgar, 1 minute	amanota umwana avukana kumunota
Neonatal	Breathing effort: If the infant is not breathing-score is 0. If the respirations are slow or irregular-score is 1. If the infant cries well-score is 2.	guhema ninguvu
Neonatal	Heart rate evaluated by stethoscope. If there is no heartbeat-score is 0. If the heart rate is less than 100 beats per minute-score is 1. If the heart rate is over 100 beats per minute-score is 2.	gupima urugero umutima utererako
Neonatal	Muscle tone. If the muscles are loose and floppy-score is 0. If there is some tone-score is 1. If there is active motion-score is 2.	ubukomezi bwimitsi
Neonatal	Grimace response or reflex irritability in response to a mild pinch. If there is no reaction-score is 0. If there is grimacing-score is 1. If there is grimacing and a cough, sneeze, or vigorous cry-score is 2.	ugukerebuka kw umwana
Neonatal	Skin color: If the color is pale blue-score is 0. If the body is pink and the extremities blue-score 1. If the entire body is pink-score is 2.	isura y urukoba
Neonatal	Apgar at 5minutes	Amanota y umwana inyuma y iminota5
Neonatal	Fontanelle	uruhoriori
GU	circumcision?	isubu?
GU	genital herpes?	umugera wo mu gitsina
GU	testicular exam	gupima amagara
Rectal	hemorrhoids,nodules, prostate on rectal exam	gupima indwara zo mu gisusu

Physical exam	English	Kirundi
Rectal	"I want to check your rectum for hemorrhoids. This might be uncomfortable. Bend over please."	Ngira ndagupime indwara yo kubora imitsi yo mu gisusu.
Neurology	"Sit up please."	"vyuka wicare, ndakwinginze."
Neurology	N1 Olfactory: coffee, peppermint? "Close your eyes and tell me what you smell."	Umutsi nsoza bwenge wo mumazuru. Humiriza uce umbwira ico wumva kimoto.
Neurology	N2 Optic: Snellen chart confrontation. "Read the letters on this chart. Follow my finger with your eyes, without moving your head."	Umutsi nsoza bwenge wo mu maso. Soma izi ndome kurizi dosiye. Kurikira intoke zanje namaso yawe, utarinze guhindukiza umutwe.
Neurology	N3,4,6 Oculomotor, Trochlear, Abducens. EOM's "Follow my finger."	Imitsi nsoza bwenge yo mu maso. "Kurikira urutoke rwanje"
Neurology	N5 Trigeminal "Clench your jaw." "Move your jaw back and forth."	Umutsi nsoza bwenge rugira 5. "Shira inguvu mu matama, hindukiza imbere n inyuma amatama yawe"
Neurology	Ophthalmic branch: forehead, Maxillary branch: cheek, Mandibular branch: chin, "Do you feel this?"	cheek = itama, chin= urusagusagu
Neurology	N7 Facial: "Raise your eyebrows."	umutsi nsoza wenge w indwi. "Hindukiza amaso yawe."
Neurology	"Close your eyes tightly, smile big."	"Humiriza, twenga cane."
Neurology	N8 Acoustic: whisper, Rinne "Can you hear me talking? Try to repeat what I say."	umutsi nsoza bwenge ugira umunani, wo kwumva. Sifura, uranyumva ndiko ndavuga? Gerageza gusubiramwo ivyo ndiko ndavuga.
Neurology	"Tell me when you can't feel the vibration."	"Urambarira nihagera ko utumva uriko uratetemera."
Neurology	N9 Glossopharyngeal: swallow (hoarseness?) "Swallow please."	Umutsi nsoza bwenge w icenda, wo kuurimi no mu magage. "Mira."
Neurology	N10 Vagus: swallow, soft palate, gag reflex "Open your mouth widely. Stick out your tongue please. Now, close it."	umutsi nsoza bwenge w icumi. Mira. "Asama cane. Sohora ururimi, ugara umunwa ubu nyene."
Neurology	N11 Spinal accessory nerve: "Turn your head to the right, now to the left. Shrug your shoulders.(like this)"	Umutsi nsoza bwenge wuruti rw umugongo. "Hindukiza umutwe urabe iburyo, hama ibubamfu. Duza ibitugu nkuku."
Neurology	N12 Hypoglossal: tongue midline	Umutsi nsoza bwenge w icumi na kabiri, wo kururimi.
Neurology	Glasgow coma score	Igipimo c ubwenge ku barwayi b indembe

Physical exam	English	Kirundi
Neurology	Opens eyes to: spontaneous (4), to speech (3), to pain (2), none (1)	kanura: bukebuke 4, bakuvugishije 3, bakubabaje 2, ntanyishu 1
Neurology	Best motor: "Hold up two fingers" obeys commands (6), localizes:reaches for the part of the body being stimulated (5), withdraws (4), abnormal flexion (3), abnormal extension (2), none (1)	ugukora neza kw imitsi: fata ugumye intoke zibiri. Yubahiriza amabwirizwa 6, Erekana neza igice cumubiri kiriko kirakorwako 5, ajana ahatariho? 4, apfunya nabi 3, agorora nabi 2, ntanyishu 1
Neurology	Best verbal: oriented (5), confused (4), inappropriate (3), garbled (2), none (1)	Kwishura ibibazo: Avuga ibitomoye 5, arihenda 4, ibitajanye 3, ibitatomoye 2, ntanyishu 1
Neurology	Motor function	Ikoreshwa ry imitsi
Neurology	biceps brachii, elbow flexion "Pull your arm up, like this."	umutsi wo kukuboko urimwo ibiri, gupfunya inkokora, duza ukuboko ukogorore, nkuku!
Neurology	wrist extensors "Bend your wrist up, like this."	gorora igikonjo. Pfunya igikonjo, nkuku!
Neurology	triceps brachii, elbow extension "Straighten your arm out, like this."	umutsi wo kukuboko urimwo itatu, gorora mu nkokora. Gorora ukuboko kwawe, nkuku!
Neurology	finger flexors, distal phalanx middle finger "bend the tip of this finger"	imitsi ipfunya intoke, uwutuma urutoke rwo hagati tupfunya
Neurology	finger abduction, little finger "hold the small finger tightly. (Don't let me squeeze your fingers together.)"	umutsi wo gupfunya agatoke kanyuma. Fata neza agatoke kanyuma.
Neurology	iliopsoas, hip flexors "Move this knee to your chest, now the other knee."	imitsi yo gupfunya amatako. Duza ivi urikoze mu gikiriza, iryiburyo, niry ibubamfu.
Neurology	quadriceps, knee extensors "Straighten your leg out, like this."	imitsi igorora amavi igizwe n imitsi 4. gorora ukuguru kwawe, nkuku!
Neurology	tibialis anterior, ankle dorsiflexors "Pull your foot up, like this."	umutsi wo kumurundi. Duza ikirenge cawe, nkuku!
Neurology	extensor hallucis longus, long toe extension "Raise your toe up, like this."	imitsi yo kugororora amano
Neurology	gastrocnemius, ankle plantar flexors "Push your foot down against my hand, like this."	imitsi yo kukirenge. Sunika niguvu ikirenge cawe mu kiganza canje, nkuku!
Neurology	"Is the sensation dull or sharp? Say sharp or dull."	wumva hameze gute?
Neurology	C-4 (top of acromioclavicular joint)	kurutugu
Neurology	C-5 (lateral side of antecubital fossa)	kukuboko
Neurology	C-6 (thumb)	urukumu

Physical exam	English	Kirundi
Neurology	C-7 (middle finger)	nsumbazose
Neurology	C-8 (little finger)	uruhererezi
Neurology	T-4 (nipple line)	kumurongo wibere
Neurology	T-10 (umbilicus)	kumukondo
Neurology	L-2 (mid-anterior thigh)	imbere hagati kwitako
Neurology	L-3 (medial femoral condyle)	hagati kwigufa ryo mwitako
Neurology	L-4 (medial malleolus)	mujisho ry ikirenge
Neurology	L-5 (dorsum of the foot, at third MTP joint)	jejuru yikirenge, mungingo igira gatatu y amano
Neurology	S-1 (Lateral heel)	hagati kugatsintsiri
Neurology	S-2 (popliteal fossa of the knee, in the midline)	muntege
Neurology	S-3 (ischial tuberosity)	mukiyunguyungu
Neurology	S4-5 (perianal area)	kugisusu
Neurology	Reflexes; "I am going to tap you here with this reflex hammer."	gupima imitsi nsozabwenge. "Ngira ndagukubite ngaha ninyundo yo kwa muganga"
Neurology	triceps right and left	initsi irimwo itatu, iburyo n ibubamfu
Neurology	biceps, right and left	umutsi urimwo ibiri, iburyo n ibubamfu
Neurology	brachioradial, right and left	imitsi yukuboko, ibubamfu niburyo
Neurology	patella, right and left	pia ya mguu; iyitfu m'ivi
Neurology	ankle, right and left	Ijisho ry ikirenge. Iburyo n ibubamfu
Neurology	babinski, right and left (great toe extension= positive)	mu kirenge, iburyo n ibubamfu
Neurology	**Tandem walk** "Walk like this, one foot in front of other." (Or, say walk like this and demonstrate.)	"tambuka nkuku!"
Neurology	**heel walk, toe walk** "Walk on your heels, now walk on your toes."	"tambukira kugatsintsiri, ubu naho tambukira kumano"
Neurology	**romberg** "Stand up, hold your arms out, close your eyes."	"haguruka.rekura amaboko,ugara amaso"
Neurology	**rapid alternating movement** (2nd finger, thumb) "Do this, fast".	gupima ubushobozi bw imitsi naningoga. Ukoresheje agakokorabukoko n urukumu. "Gira nkuku, ningoga!"
Neurology	**heel-shin** "Close your eyes. Move your right heel from your left knee to the ankle. Now, move your left heel from your right knee down to the ankle." (Open your eyes, let me demonstrate.)	"ugara amaso. shira agatsintsiri kiburyo kwivi, ukamanure ugashikane kujisho ryikirenge. Gira ibubamfu nkuku nyene. Kanura, reka ndabikwereke"
Neurology	**finger nose finger** "Touch my finger with your finger then touch your nose."	urutoke iyuru urutoke. "Kora kurutoke rwanje nurutoke rwawe hama wikore kuzuru"

Physical exam	English	Kirundi
Neurology	**stereognosis** (key, pencil, cup) "Close your eyes; what is this in your hand?"	Kumeya ibikoresho nintoke utakoresheje amaso. "Urufunguruzo, ikaramu yigiti, igikombe. Humiriza, iki nigiki kiri mu minwe yawe?"
Neurology	**graphesthesia** (draw #3 in hand) "Close your eyes, what is the number written in your hand?"	Kumenya ico bakwanditseko utakibonye. "Capa #3 mukiganza. Nikihe giharuro nanditse mukiganza cawe?"
Neurology	**point localization**: "Close your eyes, tell me what part of your body is being touched."	kumenya igihimba cawe bakozeko utakibonye. "Humiriza, mbarirw igihimba cawe nakozeko"
Neurology	**two point discrimination**: "Do you feel one or two points of contact?"	ibice bibiri bikozweko/."wumva igihimba kimwe canke ibihimba bibiri nakozeko?"
Mental status	SLUMS Examination	Igipimo c urugero rw ubwenge
Mental status	Saint Louis University Mental Status Examination	
Mental status	What day of the week is it? (1)	Turi kumunsi wakangahe wo mundwi?
Mental status	What is the year? (1)	Turi mu mwaka wa kangahe?
Mental status	What state are we in? (1)	Turi mukihe gisagara?
Mental status	Please remember these five objects. I will ask you what they are later. Pineapple Pen Hat House Car	Ndagusavye wibuke ibi bikoresho bitanu. Ndaza kubikubaza hanyuma. Inanasi, Ikaramu, Inkofero, Inzu, Imodoka
Mental status	You have 1000 francs and you go to the store and buy a dozen mangoes for 300 francs and fabric for 200francs. How much did you spend? (1) How much do you have left? (2)	Ufise amafaranga 1000 yo muri kongo hama uce uja kugur Imyembe yamajana atatu, nigitambara c amajana abiri. Wakoresheje amafaranga angahe?1 Usigaranye angahe?2
Mental status	Please name as many animals as you can in one minute. (0) 0-4 animals, (1) 5-9 animals, (2) 10-14 animals, (3) 15+ animals	ndagusavye uvuge amazina y ibikoko menshi ushoboye mumunota umwe: i 0. ibikoko 0_4, 1. ibikoko 5_9, 2. ibikoko 10_14, 3. ibikoko birenga 15
Mental status	What were the five objects I asked you to remember? pineapple Pen Tie House Car. One point for each correct answer.	Nibihe bikoresho bitanu nagusavye ngo uze kwibuka? Inanasi, Ikaramu, Ikaruvati, inzu, imodoka. Inota rimwe kunyishu imwimwe nziza.
Mental status	I am going to give you a series of numbers and I would like you to give them to me backwards. For example, if I say 42, you say 24. (0) 87, (1) 649, (2) 8537	Ngira ndaguhe urutonde rwibiharuro hama ndagusaba ko nawe uza kubisubiramwo hanyuma. Akarorero: mvuze 42, uca wishura 24. (0). 87,(1) 649, (2) 8537
Mental status	This is a clock face. Please put in the hour markers and the time at ten minutes to eleven o'clock. (2) Hour markers correct? (2) Time correct?	Iyi n isaha. Shiramwo ibimenyetso vy amasaha, hama werekane sa tanu zibura iminota icumi. (2) yabikoza neza, (2) Umwanya mwiza?

30

Physical exam	English	Kirundi
Mental status	Place an X in the triangle. □△◇, (1) Which of the figures is the largest? (1)	Shira uyu musaraba munyabutatu 1. nikihe gicapo kinini muri ibi? 1
Mental status	I am going to read you a story. Please listen carefully because afterwards, I'm going to ask you some questions about it. Jill was a very successful doctor. She made a lot of money on the stock market. She then met Jack, a strong man. She married him and had three children. They lived in Goma. She then stopped work and stayed at home to bring up her children. When they were teenagers, she went back to work. She and Jack lived happily ever after.	ngira ndagutere inkuru. Ndagusavye wumvirize neza kuko mpejeje ndaza kukubaza utubazo. Jill yari umuganga afise umugisha, yararonka amafaranga menshi mukuvura abantu. Hama ahura na Yakobo, umugabo akomeye cane. Barakungana hama barubakana, hama bavyara abana batatu. baba igoma. Hama aca ahagarika gukora, aja kurera abana. bamaze kugera mu bigeo, aca asubira kukazi. Hama we na Yakobo baca baribanira akaramata.
Mental status	What was the female's name? (2)	Umugore yitwa gute? 2
Mental status	What work did she do? (2)	yakora iki? 2
Mental status	When did she go back to work? (2)	yasubiye kukazi ryari? 2
Mental status	What state did she live in? (2)	yaba mukihe gisagara? 2
Mental status	Add total score, with high school education: 27-30 normal, 21-26 mild cognitive disorder, 1-20 dementia. Without high school education: 25-30 normal, 20-24 mild cognitive disorder, 1-19 dementia.	teranya amanota yose. Kuwize kaminuza: 27_30 bimeza neza, 21_26 afise indwara ikiri nto, 1_20 ararwaye cane. Kuwutize amashuri menshi: 25_30 bimeza neza. 20_24 arwaye bukebuke, 1_19 ararwaye cane

Joint exam	English	Kirundi
	Shoulder test for impingement. Apley scratch test: Use your right hand to touch the left scapula by reaching over the left clavicle. Next, use your right hand to touch the right scapula. Thirdly, move your right thumb to the middle of your back between the scapulae. "Move your arm like I do"	Gupima Igitugu. Apley scratch test: ukoresheje ukuboko kwawe kwiburyo, kora kwigufa ryigitugu ibubamfu ucishije ukuboko imbere yizosi. Hama, ukoresheje ukuboko kwiburyo kora kwigufa ryurutugu rwiburyo. Ubwa gatatu, koza urutoke rwurukumu rwawe mumugongo hagati yogufa ryurutugu. (Kurikiza ukwo ndiko ndagira)
	Shoulder test for impingement.Neers test: Place one hand on the patient's scapula, grasp their forearm with your other hand (their thumb should be facing down). Slowly forward flex the arm. "I am going to put my hand on your shoulder blade and move your arm."	Gupima igitugu. Neers Test: shira ukuboko kumwe kwigufa ryurutugu rwumurwayi, cufata amaboko yabo (Urabisha intoke zinkumu zabo hasi). Ca urekura bukebuke ukuboko. " Ngira nshire ikiganzacanje kurutugu rwawe hama nce nduza ukuboko kwawe."
	Supraspinatus isometric test: the patient holds their arm at 20 degrees abduction and the examiner attempts adduction. "Hold your arm like this and try to raise it."	Supraspinatus isometric test: umurwayi ashira amaboko imbere kuri degre 20, hama umuganga akagerag16za kuyasubiza inyuma (shira ukuboko kwawe ngaha, hama ugerageze kukugumizayo)
	Supraspinatus function. Painful arc sign: "I am going to raise your arm, let me know when you have pain."	Supraspinatus function. Painful arc sign: ngira nduze ukuboko kwawe, urambarira niwumva ubabaye
	Supraspinatus function. Drop arm test: raise the arm to 180 degrees abduction then instruct the patient: "Slowly lower your arm to your side". If the arm falls quickly the test is positive.	Supraspinatus function. Drop arm test: duza ukuboko imbere ushikane kuri degre 180 hama usigurire umurwayi: Manutse bukebuke ukuboko kwawe, ukwiyegerezako. Ukuoko nikwarwa ningoga naningoga igipimo kiba cerekanye indwara
	Tinel test for ulnar nerve entrapment: tap over the ulnar groove and ask "Do you have pain or numbness. If so, show me where it hurts?" (Pain and numbness at 4th, 5th fingers indicates a positive test.)	"Urababara ngaha?" Korako n urutoke aho wumva ubabara.
	Phalen maneuver for carpal tunnel syndrome: hold the wrist in forced flexion. Pain is a positive indication. "Do you have pain, where?"	"Urababara ngaha, hehe?"

Joint exam	English	Kirundi
	Scaphoid compression test. The thumb is held and pushed toward the scaphoid. Pain indicates a possible scaphoid fracture. **"Do you feel pain."**	**"Urababara ngaha?"**
	Hip assessment. Perform internal and external rotation of the hip and ask, **"Does this hurt?"**	**"Urababara ngaha?"**
	Piriformis test Patient is in lateral decubitus position with hip flexed at 60 degrees and knee at full extension. Examiner places a hand on the patient's shoulder and exerts mild pressure on the flexed leg at the knee. A positive test is noted by radicular pain caused by impingement of the sciatic nerve by the tight piriformis muscle. **"Lay on your left side, and now, lay on your right side."**	**"Ryamira urubavu rw ukubamfu. Ryamira urubavu rw iburyo."**
	Ely's test to assess rectus femoris flexibility. Patient lays prone with legs fully extended. Examiner passively flexes the knee to full ROM. If the ipsilateral hip rises it is suggestive of a tight rectus femoris muscle. **"Lay on your abdomen."**	**"Ryama wubitse inda."**
	Fulcrum test Patient is seated on a table with legs dangling. Examiner places their forearm under the thigh for use as a fulcrum. Pressure is applied with the other hand over the knee and up the femur. Pain elicited may indicate a stress fracture. **"Sit on the edge of the bed."**	**"Vyuka, icara aha."**
	Straight leg raise **"Lay down, I am going to lift your leg, let me know where you feel pain."**	Duza ukuguru. **"Ryama hasi, ngira nduze ukuguru kwawe, urambarira wumvise umusonga"**
	Knee collateral ligament assessment. valgus stress for medial instability. **"Lay down. I am going to check your knee."** Place one hand on lateral thigh while the other hand is used to apply outward pressure on the calf.	**Gupima imitsi yo mu mavi "Ryama hasi, ngira mpime ivi ryawe"**
	Knee collateral ligament assessment. varus stress for lateral instability **"Lay down. I am going to check your knee."** Place one hand on the medial thigh while the other hand is used to apply inward pressure on the calf.	**Gupima imitsi yo mu mavi:" Ryama hasi, ngira mpime ivi ryawe"**
	Lachman's test for anterior cruciate ligament injury (ACL) **"Lay down, bend your knee."** Place the knee at 30 degrees flexion, stabilize the the femur with one hand while pulling the proximal tibia anteriorly. Laxity indicates ACL injury.	**"Ryama hasi ugaramye, pfunya ivi ryawe"**
	Pivot shift test for ACL injury. **"Lay down."** With the knee in full extension the examiner rotates the tibia and applies valgus stress then flexes the knee. If acl injury is present a "clunk" sound will be heard.	**"Ryama ugaramye".**

33

Joint exam	English	Kirundi
	Anterior drawer for ACL injury. **"Lay down and bend your knee."** to 90 degrees. The examiner hold the proximal tibia with both hands, sits on the patient's foot and pulls the tibia anteriorly to look for laxity.	**"Ryama hasi ugaramye, pfunya ivi ryawe."**
	Posterior drawer test for posterior cruciate ligament injury (PCL) Patient is supine with the hips flexed at 45 degrees and knees at 90 degrees, Examiner sits on the patient's feet, grasps the tibia with both hands and applies backward pressure. Laxity is a sign of a torn posterior cruciate ligament. **"Lay on your back and bend your knee."**	**"Ryama ugaramye, pfunya ivi ryawe".**
	Thessaly test: for knee meniscal injury**"Stand up. Bend your knee and then turn it like this(move your leg like I do)."** Patient should hold the examiner's hand, stand on one leg with the knee flexed at 20 degrees. The patient then internally and externally rotates their knees. Pain or locking is a positive test.	**"Haguruka. Pfunya ivi. (Hindukiza ukuguru nkuko ngize)"**
	Apley test for knee meniscal injury **"Lay on your abdomen."** With patient prone bend the knee to 90 degrees and apply downward pressure while internally and externally rotating the foot. Pain indicates a positive test.	**"Ryama wubitse inda."**
	Ottawa knee rules X ray indicated if any of following are present: 1. age over 55 "What is your age?" 2. Tenderness of patella: "Do you have pain here?" 3. Tenderness of fibular head: "Do you have pain here." Inability to flex the knee to 90 degrees: "4. Bend your knee as much as possible." 5. Inability to transfer weight to each leg. "Stand on your right leg only, now on your left leg only."	**1. Ufise imyaka ingahe? 2. Ububabare hano? 3. Ububabare hano? 4. Pfunya ivi, cane. 5. Haguruka, ukuguru kw'iburyo, ukuguru kw'ibubamfu."**
	Ottawa ankle rules, part 1. An ankle x ray is indicated if there is inability to bear weight in the ER or there is tenderness at the posterior edge or tip of the medial or lateral malleolus (distal 6cm). **"Can you walk? Do you have pain when I touch here?"**	**"Uragenda? Urababara ngaha?"**
	Ottawa ankle rules, part 2. A foot x ray is indicated if there is inability to bear weight in the ER or there is tenderness at the base of the 5th metatarsal or over the navicular bone. **"Can you walk? Do you have pain when I touch here?"**	**"Uragenda? Urababara ngaha?"**

Joint exam	English	Kirundi
	Thompson test for achilles tendon rupture. The patient lays prone with their feet hanging over the end of the bed. The calf muscles are squeezed and if the Achilles tendon is ruptured there is no plantar flexion of the foot.**"Lay on your abdomen."**	**"Ryama wubitse inda."**

Counseling	English	Kirundi
Emergency	Go to the emergency room if you: 1) cough or vomit blood, 2) break a bone 3) have sudden severe illness 4) have numbness in your face, legs or arms 5) are severely burned 6) injure your head 7) have an injured infant.	Genda gukoresha icumba cakira abaremvya ni: 1) ukorora kandi udahwa amaraso 2) wavunika igufa 3) wagize ingwara, giturumbuka, 4) wumva itiyumva mu maso, ku maguru, canke ku maboko 5) wahiye (ubushe) bikomeye cane 6) wakomeretse ku mutwe 7) umwana wawe yakomeretse
	Go to the emergency room if you have: 1) chest pain or trouble speaking 2) high fever with stiff neck, mental confusion or trouble breathing 3) severe shortness of breath (gasping for air) 4) poisoning 5) sudden loss of consciousness	Genda gukoresha icumba cakira abaremvya ni: 1) ubabara cane mugikiriza, canke wagize ingorane zokuvuga 2) Ufise umuriro mwinshi manwe n'izosi ridadaraye, wumva uriko urata ubwenge, canke ufise ingorane zoguhema 3) wagize ingorane zoguhema zirengeje urugero (ubura impemu) 4) iyo wariye ishano 5)uta ubwenge giturumbuka
Pulmonary	You need to go for an x ray.	Genda mw'iradio.
	I have the result of your sputum.	Ndafise inyishu zibipimo y igikororwa canyu.
	You have...	Murafise.....
	tuberculosis	igitintu
	pneumonia	Indwara y amahaha
	Your lungs are affected, you need to quit smoking today.	Amahaha yanyu aradwaye, mutegerezwa guhagarika kuywa itabi kuva uyu munsi.
	You must stop smoking.	Mutegerezwa guhagarika kunywa itabi
Cardiac	Avoid smoking or being around people that smoke.	Irinde kunywa itabi n'ukwegera abarinywa.
	Limit alcoholic drinks.	Igerer mu binyobwa.
	Don't get too fat.	Wirinde kuvyibuha cane.
	Signs of a heart attack include:	Ibimenyetso vy'indwara y'umutima:
	Pain in the center of the chest that lasts more than a few minutes or that goes away and comes back	Ububabare hagati mu gikiriza bumara umwanya muto canke buza begenda bwongera bugaruka.
	pain in one or both arms, the back, neck, jaw or stomach.	Ubababare mu kuboko kumwe canke mu maboko yose, mu mugongo, kw'izosi, mu musaya canke, mu mushishito.
	Shortness of breath with or without chest pain.	Guhema udashikana (ignorane mu guhema, canke mugusama impemu) ubabara canke utababara mu gikiriza.
	Breaking out in a cold sweat, nausea or feeling faint.	Gufatwa bukumbi n'intuguta y'icuya gikonje, kugira isesem canke kwumva uyamira nk'uwuzunguriwe.

Counseling	English	Kirundi
Neurologic	Signs of a stroke include:	Ibimenyetso vy'indwara y'ubwonko iterwa n'iziba ry'imitsi itwara amaraso mu bwonko:
	Sudden numbness or weakness of the face, arm or leg, especially on one side of the body.	Uruhande rumwe ry'umubiri, ukuguru kumwe, ukuboko kumwe, uruhande rw'umunwa hamwe n'ijisho rimwe riherereye kuri urwo ruhande birapfa.
	Trouble speaking or understanding	Ingorane yo kuvuga no gutergera ibivuzwe.
	Trouble seeing with one or both eyes.	Ingorane yo kubonesha ijisho rimwe canke yose.
	Trouble walking, dizziness or loss of balance or coordination.	Ingorane yo gutambuka, kuzungurirwa, hamwe no gushobora guhagarara neza udahenuka.
	Sudden severe headache with no known cause.	Ukumeneka/ukubabara mu mutwe bishika giturumbuka, ata mpuamvu zizwi zihari.
Infectious disease	You are sick with malaria.	Murarwaye Inyonko.
	You have typhoid fever.	Murarwaye tifoyide.
	You have intestinal worms.	Murarwaye inzoka zo munda.
	It will take time for you to heal.	Bizogufata umwanya kugire ngo ukire.
	HIV can be transmitted through blood, semen, and vaginal secretions.	Umugera wa SIDA wandukira biciye mu maraso, m'umbuto z'umugabo, mu maberebere no mu ruziri ruva mubihimba vy'irondoka vy'umugore, vy'abantu banduye uwo mugera wa SIDA.
	HIV cannot be transmitted by: 1)casual contact 2)shaking hands 3)hugging,kissing 4) cough,sneezing 5) giving blood 6)sitting on toilet seats 7) sharing bed linen 8) sharing forks, spoons, knives, plates bowls or glasses 9) mosquito or other insect bites	Ntushobora kwandura umugera wa SIDA mugukora ibikurikira: 1) gukoranako bisanzwe 2) kuramukanya n'amaboko 3)kurwana w'unda 4) gukorra, kwasamura 5) gutanga amaraso 6) kwicara ku kazu kasugumwe kikizungu 7) gusangira amashuka 8) gusangira amafurusheti ibiyiko, imbugita, amasahani, amabakure canke ibirahuri 9) kuribwa n'imibu canke n'utundi dukoko turyana
Gastroenterology	There is an ulcer in your stomach.	Murafise indwara ya iriseri yo mumushishito.
	You need to quit drinking beer completely.	Mutegerezwa guhagarika kunywa inzoga burundu.
	You have a tumor in your stomach.	Murafise ikivyimba mu mushishito.
	I need to put a suppository in your rectum.	Nagira nshire ikinini mu gisusu canyu.
	The symptoms of hepatitis B include: 1) weakness and tiredness 2) loss of appetite 3) nausea or vomiting 4) diarrhea or constipation 5) dark urine 6) fever 7) headache 8) itchy skin 9)joint pain and rashes.	Iimenyetso vy'indwara y'igitigu bishobora kuba: 1) intege nke n'ukuruha 2) ugutakaza akayabagu 3) ugusesemewa n'nkudabwa 4) ugucibwamwo n'ukutaja kwituma 5)amasobe yirabura 6) inyonko 7) ukurneneka umutwe 8) ukubabswa ku rukoba 9) ubabare bwo mu ngingo n'uruhere

37

Counseling	English	Kirundi
Surgery	We need to take you to surgery.	Turifuza kubatwara mu cumba co kubagirwamo.
	When have you last eaten?	Muheruka kufungura ryari.
	Have you eaten in the last six hours?	Harico mwafunguye mu masaha atandatu aheze?
	Do not eat or drink until after surgery.	Ntihagire ico munywa canke ngo mufungure, imbere ninyuma yo kubarwa.
	I need to have sew up (suture) this wound.	Ngire ndagushone aha kugikomere.
	You are badly injured.	Wakomeretse cane.
	The operation went very well.	Igikorwa co kukubaga cagenze neza .
	You need to stay in bed.	Mutegerezwa kuguma mugitanda.
	You need to stay in the hospital.	Mutegerezwa kuguma mu bitaro.
	I need to change your dressing.	Nifuza kubahindurira ivyambarwa.
Pharmacy	I will give you medication.	Ndaza kuguha umuti.
	This medicine is for pain.	Uyu muti nuwububabare.
	This medicine is for the infection.	Uyu muti ni uwa ifection.
	Do not drink alcohol while on this medicine.	Ntihagire inzoga munywa mukiriko murafata uyu muti.
	You take this medicine a) once b) two, c) three, d)four times per day.	Mufata uy muti a)Rimwe b)Kabiri c)Gatatu, d) Kane kumunsi
	Take this medicine until the bottle is empty.	Murafata uyu muti gushika muwumaze.
	Take this medication twice a day only if you need to.	Murafata uyu mutikabiri kumunsi iyo bikenewe.
	Take this medication before eating.	Murafata uyu muti imbere yo gufungura.
	Take this medication with food.	Murafata uyu muti, muriko murafungura.
	Take this medication on an empty stomach.(an hour before or two hours after a meal)	Murafata uyu muti ataco murafungura (Isaha imwe imbere yo gufungura canke isaha zibiri muhejeje gufungura)
	Take this medicine a) each morning b) each night.	Murafata uyu muti a)burimunsi mugatondo b) buri munsi mwijoro
	Take this medicine for a) one week, b) for one (1), two (2), three (3) days.	Murafata uyu muti a)Indwi imwe, b) umunsi umwe c)iminsi ibiri d)iminsi itatu.
	Take this medication after meals.	Murafata uyu muti iyo muhejeje gufungura.
	Take this medication in the morning.	Murafata uyu muti mugatondo.
	Take this medication at night.	Murafata uyu muti mwijoro.
	This medicine may change the color of your urine.	Uyu muti uzohindura ibara ry umukoyo wanyu.

Counseling	English	Kirundi
	Do not take this with dairy products.	Ntihagire ikintu kindi muzofatana nuyu muti.
	Place drops in your bad ear.	Murakororera amama yuyu muti mugutwi kurwaye.
	Unwrap and insert one suppository in your rectum.	Murugurura hama mushire ikinini mu gisusu.
	Spray this in your nose.	Murapuriza uyu muti mumazuru.
	Inhale by mouth (like this).	Hemera mukanwa (Nkuku).
	Insert the suppository into your vagina.	Murashira iki kinini mubihimba vyirondoka (polite form, names of genital parts sound impolite in kirundi)
	Place drops in this eye.	Murashira amama yuyu muti muri iri jisho.
Maternity/Ob	Congratulations, you are pregnant!	Nezerwa, Uribungenze!
	The baby is due on this date...	Muzokwibaruka kwitariki......
	Take a daily multivitamin or a vitamin with 400micrograms of folic acid.	Fata ikinini ca multivitamine ku munsi ku munsi canka vitamine B6 ifasha abari mu kwibaruka (400mcg ya folic acid)
	During the prenatal visit the nurse midwife or doctor will:	Mu gihe uja kuraba abaganga witagurira kwibaruka, muganga:
	Do a complete physical exam, including a pelvic exam and pap smear.	Azosuzuma ibihimba vy'umbubiri vyinshi, harimwo gusuzuma ingene amaguta akikije igitereko ameze (pelvis) n'urwinjirero rw'igitereko c'umukenyezi.
	Take blood and urine.	Azogufata amaraso hamwe n'amasobwa
	Check blood pressure, height and weight.	Azopima umurindi w'amaraso, uburebure, n'ibiro ufise.
	Calculate the due date, a date near which the baby will be born.	Azoharura umunsi uzokwibarukirako, italiki yegereje igihe umwana azotegerezwa kuba yavukiyeko.
	Check the baby's heart rate.	Azopima ingene umutima w'umwana wibugenze utera.
	Signs of trouble during pregnancy: If you are bleeding bright red blood or blood is soaking through your underwear, go to the hospital immediately.	Ibimenyetso bishobora kuba bitara ingorane: Ni waba uva amaraso atukura rwose canka amaraso akaba acafuza ikaleso yawa, genda kwa mugnga mu maguru masha.
	At 16 weeks of pregnancy, your baby should move 10 times within two hours every day. If you baby is not moving this much after 1-2 hours, contact the doctor.	Kuva ku ndwi ya 16 wibungenze, uruyoya rwawa rwotegerezwa kwihindukiza agashika 10 uko amasasha abiri aheze. Ni rwaba uruyoya rwawe n'ubu rudakakaza inyuma y'isasha imwe canke amasaha abiri, hamagara muganga.
	The nurse is on her way.	Umu foroma araje.
	She will help with the delivery.	Aragufasha kwibaruka.
	You had a boy. You had a girl.	Mwibarutse Umuhungu. Mwibarutse umukobwa.
	You had twins.	Mwibarutse Amahasa.

39

Counseling	English	Kirundi
	You will need a cesarean section.	Bategerezwa kukubaga.
Women's health	Birth control options include:	Uburyo bwo gukinga gutwara inda:
	condoms: condoms are placed over the penis before intercourse. Condoms are the only type of birth control that also protects against sexually transmitted diseases like HIV/ AIDS. There are condoms made for men and women.	Udufuko: udufuko batwambika igihimba c'irondoka c'umugabo imbere yo kurangura amabanga y'irondoka. Udufuko ni bwo buryo bwonyene bukinga gutwara inda kandi bugakinga ingwara zifatira mu bihimba vy'irondoka nka SIDA. Hari ubwoko bubuir bw'udufuko; kamwe 'kabagore n'akabagabo.
	Oral contraceptives: This birth control pill is for women to swallow by mouth. It is taken daily.	Ibinini vyo kumira: ubwo buryo ni ikinini abagore bamira bacishije mu kanwa. Ico kinini n'ukukimira buri munsi.
	Depo-vera injection: this birth control is injected like a shot to the woman every 3 months.	Inshinge bita depo-vera injections: ubwo buryo ni umuti batera mu mubiri nk'urushinge rusanzwe uko amezi 3 aheze.
	Novaring: this birth control is in the shape of a ring and is inserted into the vagina. It is worn for three weeks and taken out while the woman is menstruating. After each menstrual cycle a new ring is used.	Uburyo bita Nuvaring: nuvaring ni akantu kameze nk'impeta umugore yiyinjizamwo mu gihimba c'irondoka. Ako kantu akigumizamwo amayinga atatu hanyuma akagakurayo mu gihe ari mu butinyanka. Iyo avuye mu butinyanka araheza agakoresha akandi gashasha.
	Intrauterine device (IUD): this birth control is a T-shaped device placed inside the woman's womb by her doctor.	Uburyo bita intrauterine device (IUD): ubu buryo bita "IUD" ni akantu karneze n'indome T umuganga ashira mu gitereko c'umugore.
	Diaphragm (cervical cap): this birth control is in the shape of a cup and placed inside the vagina before sexual intercourse.	Uburyo bita diaphragm/cervical cap. Ivyo bita "diaphragm/cervical cap" ni akantu kameze nk'agakombe umugore yinjiza mu gihimba c'irondoka imbere yo kurangura amabanga y'abubatse.
	Tubal ligation: this birth control is a surgery done on women. It is a permanent method of birth control for women who decide never to have children again.	Uburya bita "tubal ligation": tubal ligation ni uburyo bukoreshwa ku bagore babanje kubabaga. Bituma umugore ahagarika gusama ubutagisubira ku buryo abavyemeye baba biyemeje kutazokwigera barondoka canke ngo basubire kuvyara abandi bana.
Procedures	"I need to take a blood sample."	Ngira ndabafate amaraso.
	"Please give me a urine sample in this cup."	Mumpe umukoyo wanyu.
	I need to put a tube in your bladder to drain the urine.	Ngire nshire akaringoti mukaziba kinda, nkureyo umukoyo.
	"Please give me a stool specimen in this container."	Murashira umusarani wanyu muri aka gacupa.
	"Please give me a sputum sample in this cup."	Murashira igikororwa canyu muri aka gacupa.

Counseling	English	Kirundi
	"I need to put this tube in your nose-it will go into your stomach"	Ngire nshire aka karingoti mu mushishito wanyu, ndagacishije muzuru.
	"This tube will drain your stomach."	Aka karingoti karavoma amazi yo mumushishito wanyu.
	"You need to swallow to help the tube go in."	Mutegerezwa kumira kugira aka karingoti karengane.
	"I need to put a tube in your chest."	Ngire nshire akaringoti mu gikiriza canyu.
	"This tube will drain the air and fluid out of your chest."	Aka karingoti karasohora ipepu n amazi mu gikira canyu.
	"I need to start an IV."	Twifuza kubatanguza imiti yo mumutsi.
	"We need to give you fluid."	Tugire tubahe imiti yo mumutsi.
	" We need to give you blood."	Turakeneye kubaha amaraso.
	I need to give you a shot 1) in the arm, 2) in the leg	Nngire ndagutere agashinge a)mu kuboko 2)mukuguru.
Orthopedics	You need an x ray of the bone.	Murakeneye kugirisha iradiyo yiri gufa.
	You have a broken leg.	Mwavunitse ukuguru
	You have a broken ankle.	Mwavunitse kujisho ryikirenge
	You have a broken arm.	Mwavunitse ukuboko
	You have a broken wrist.	mwavunitse igikonjo
	You have fluid in your joint.	Murafise amazi mwiteranirizo ryiri gufa
	You need a cast.	Mukeneye isima
	Do not remove or get the cast wet.	Ntimuzohave mukurako canke mukanyishe iyi sima
	You may take the splint off to bathe but it must be put back on afterwards.	Murashobora gukurako aka gatambara mugiye kwoga, ariko mutegerezwa kugasubizako mugiheza.
	We need to do surgery to place a metal plate with screws to help the bone heal.	Tugire tubakore, turashira icuma mwigufa kugire turifashe gukira.
Psychiatric	You could be depressed if you have the following symptoms: 1) feel sad all the time 2) cry a lot 3) never want to go out 4) have no energy 5) sleep a lot or have difficulty sleeping	Mugabo har'aho woba ukeneye gufashwa mu gihe: 1) wama wijiriwe 2) urira cane 3) utigera ushaka kuja hanze 4) wama ukonyokewe 5) usinzira cane, canke bikugora gusinzira
	It is not healthy to feel sad all the time.	Iyo wama wijirirwe igihe cose ntuba ufise amagara meza.
	You could talk to a social worker; psychologist.	Urashobora kubiyagira n'aba: abakozi b'imibano; umugana bw'ukwiyumvira n'inyifato

Counseling	English	Kirundi
	A person may need help from a mental health worker or psychiatrist if they: 1) cannot stop being sad all the time 2) are afraid of others all the time 3) change their behavior in an unusual way 4) become violet 5) start to imagine things that are not real.	Umuntu yoba akeneye gufashwa mu bijanye n'ingwara zo mu mutwe mu gihe: 1) adashoboye kureka kwama yijiriwe 2) kwama atinya abuntu igihe cose 3) guhinduka akagira kamere kadasanzwe 4) atanguye gusinda 5) atanguye kwiyumvira ibintu bitariho
Pediatrics	Your child looks fine.	Umwana wanyu asa neza or ameze neza.
	Your child will be ill for quite a while.	Umwana wanyu azomara imins mike arwaye.
	Give the child small amounts of food every few hours.	Muraha umwana utwokurya dukeduke buri masaha make.
	Give your child this to drink every few hours.	Uyu mwana muze muramuha uyu muti uko amasaha make aheze.
	It is ok to let your child sleep.	Vyoba vyiza muretse uyu mwana agasinzira.
	Bring your child back to the clinic tomorrow.	Muragarukana uyu mwana kwa muganga ejo.
Dental	Children with tooth decay with have dental problems later in life.	Abana bafise amenyo amera asa n'ayamunzwe bashobora kugira ingorane kera mubuzima.
	Brush your child's teeth lightly with a tooth brush.	Uribuka kumwogereza amenyo ukoresheje kologati w'amuti woza amenyo.
	Brush the back and top of the front teeth. Don't forget to brush the back teeth. Brush your gums as well.	Uroza inyuma no hejuru mumenyo y'imbere. Ntukigagire kwoza arya menyo. Uroza nibinyigishi.
General	What you have is not serious.	Indwara yanyu ntabwo ikomeye cane.
	You will be better soon.	Muzogira mitende vuba.
	Don't worry, you'll get better.	Ntugire ikibazo, uzokira vuba.
	Your condition is grave.	Indwara yanyu irakomeye.
	Please come back if you have more problems.	Mugize ikibazo, muzoce mugaruka.
	Please return in one week.	Muzogaruka haheze indwi imwe.

Date/time, numbers	English	Kirundi
	January	Nzero
	February	Ruhuhuma
	March	Rubungubungu
	April	Gacabiraro
	May	Rusama
	June	Ruheshi
	July	Mukakaro
	August	Myandagaro
	September	Nyakanga
	October	Gitugutu
	November	Munyonyo
	December	Kigarama
	Sunday	kuw'Imana
	Monday	kuwa mbere
	Tuesday	kuwa kabiri
	Wednesday	kuwa gatatu
	Thursday	kuwa kane
	Friday	kuwa gatanu
	Saturday	kuwa gatandatu
	0 (zero)	zero
	1 one	rimwe
	2 two	kabiri
	3 three	gatatu
	4 four	kane
	5 five	gatanu
	6 six	gatandatu
	7 seven	indwi
	8 eight	umunani
	9 nine	icenda
	10 ten	icumi
	11 eleven	icumi n'umwe
	12 twelve	icumi na babiri
	13 thirteen	icumi na batatu
	14 fourteen	icumi na bane
	15 fifteen	icumi na batanu
	16 sixteen	icumi na batandatu
	17 seventeen	icumi n'indwi

Date/time, numbers	English	Kirundi
	18 eighteen	icumi n'umunani
	19 nineteen	icumi n'icenda
	20 twenty	mirongwibiri
	21 twenty-one	mirongwibiri n'umwe
	30 thirty	mirongwitatu
	31 thirty-one	mirongwitatu n'umwe
	40 forty	mirongwine
	50 fifty	mirongwitanu
	60 sixty	mirongwitandatu
	70 seventy	mirongwirindwi
	71 seventy-one	mirongo indwi na rimwe
	72 seventy-two	mirongo indwi na kabiri
	73 seventy-three	mirongo indwi na gatatu
	74 seventy-four	mirongo indwi na kane
	75 seventy-five	mirongo indwi na gatanu
	76 seventy-six	mirongo indwi na gatandatu
	77 seventy-seven	mirongo indwi n'indwi
	78 seventy-eight	mirongo indwi n'umunani
	79 seventy-nine	mirongo indwi n'icenda
	80 eighty	mirongwirindwi
	81 eighty-one	mirongo umunani na rimwe
	82 eighty-two	mirongo umunani na kabiri
	90 ninety	mirongwicenda
	91 ninety-one	mirongo icenda na rimwe
	92 ninety-two	mirongo icenda na kabiri
	100 one hundred	ijana
	200 two hundred	amajana abiri
	300 three hundred	amajana atatu
	400 four hundred	amajana ane
	500 five hundred	amajana atanu
	600 six hundred	amajana atandatu
	700 seven hundred	amajana indwi
	800 eight hundred	amajana umunani
	900 nine hundred	amajana icenda
	1000 one thousand	igihumbi
	1500 one thousand five hundred	igihumbi n'amajana atanu
	2000 two thousand	ibihumbi bibiri
	2500 two thousand five hundred	ibihumbi bibiri n'amajana atanu
	5000 five thousand	ibihumbi bitanu

Date/time, numbers	English	Kirundi
	At what time?	Isaha zingahe?
	At 8p.m. (this evening)	Isaha zibiri z'umugoroba.
	At noon.	Isaha zitandatu.
	It is 9 a.m.	Ni isaha zitatu.
	It is 2:30 p.m.	Ni isaha umunani z'umuhingamo.
	It is 7:15 a.m.	Ni isaha imwe n'iminata cumi n'itanu.
	It is 10:45 a.m.	Ni isha zine n'iminata mirongo ine n'itanu.
	today	uyu musi
	tomorrow	ejo
	yesterday	ejo
	soon	vuba
	right now	nonaha
	now	ubu
	morning	igitondo
	afternoon	umuhingamo
	evening	umugoroba
	night	ijoro
	last week	indwi iheze
	this week	ino ndwi
	next week	indwi iza
	last year	umwaka ukeze
	this year	uno mwaka
	next year	umwaka uza
	one week	indwi imwe
	two weeks	indwi zibiri
	one month	ukwezi kumwe
	two months	amezi abiri
	three months	amezi atatu
	four months	amezi ane
	five months	amezi atanu

Body parts	English	Kirundi
HEENT	head	umutwe
HEENT	skull	umutwe
HEENT	hair	umushatsi
HEENT	forehead	uruhanga
HEENT	face	amaso
HEENT	eye (eyes)	ijisho
HEENT	pupil	imbonero
HEENT	eyebrow (eyebrows)	ikigohe (ibigohe)
HEENT	eyelash/eyelid	urugohe (ingohe)
HEENT	nose	izuru
HEENT	nostril (nostrils)	itonde
HEENT	ear (ears)	ugutwi (amatwi)
HEENT	earlobe	igishato c'ugutwi
HEENT	tongue	ururimi
HEENT	tooth (teeth)	iryinyo
HEENT	cheek	itama
HEENT	lip (lips)	umunwa (iminwa)
HEENT	tonsils	amagage
HEENT	throat	umuhogo
HEENT	mouth	akanwa
HEENT	chin	urusagusagu; urusakanwa
HEENT	mandible	amashanya
HEENT	neck (anterior)	izosi
HEENT	adam's apple	imbeke
Upper limbs	clavicle	umugororo
Upper limbs	shoulder (shoulders)	ururtuga (intuga)
Upper limbs	axilla	ubwakwaha
Upper limbs	humerus	ikizigira
Upper limbs	arm (arms)	ukuboko
Upper limbs	upper arm	ikizigira
Upper limbs	elbow (elbows)	inkokora
Upper limbs	lower arm	ikizigira
Upper limbs	wrist	igikonjo
Upper limbs	palm of hand	ikiganza
Upper limbs	hand (hands)	ikiganza (ibiganza)
Upper limbs	thumb	urukumu
Upper limbs	finger (fingers)	urutoke (intoke)
Upper limbs	5th finger	uruhererezi
Upper limbs	4th finger	marere
Upper limbs	3rd finger	nsumbazose

46

Body parts	English	Kirundi
Upper limbs	2nd finger	nkumbaruboko
Upper limbs	knuckle	ingingo y'urutoke
Upper limbs	fingernail	urwara
Thorax	lower back	umugongo
Thorax	scapula	urushi w'ukuwoko
Thorax	chest	igikiriza
Thorax	rib (ribs)	urubavu
Thorax	heart	umutima
Thorax	lung (lungs)	ihaha (amahaha)
Thorax	breast (breasts)	ibere (amabere)
Thorax	nipples	amasonzi
Abdomen	abdomen	inda
Abdomen	esophagus	umuhogo
Abdomen	liver	igitigu
Abdomen	stomach	inda; umushishito
Abdomen	gallbladder	agasho k'indurwe
Abdomen	intestines, small	uwura w'amayoge
Abdomen	colon	umurungoro
Abdomen	rectum	umurongoro
Abdomen	spleen	urwakashya
Abdomen	kidney (kidneys)	ifigo (amafigo)
Abdomen	urethra	uruhago
Abdomen	ureter	inkaka
Abdomen	pancreas	Urwagasha
Abdomen	urinary bladder	Akaziba kinda
Abdomen	umbilicus	umukondo
Abdomen	umbilical cord	uruzogi
Pelvis	buttock (buttocks)	itako (amatako)
Pelvis	vagina	Igisundi or Igituba but not in use, sounds impolite. better is(Igihimba cirondoka)
Pelvis	clitoris	ikinena; akusino
Pelvis	uterus (womb)	intanya; igitereko
Pelvis	genitalia	ibihimba vy'irondoka
Pelvis	anus	inyo
Pelvis	penis	imboro
Pelvis	scrotum/testicle	umuruga/itengatwa
Pelvis	pelvis (groin)	urukenyerero
Pelvis	hip	umusoso
Lower limbs	femur/thigh	umuwero/ikiwero
Lower limbs	leg (legs)	ukuguru (akaguru)
Lower limbs	knee	ivi (amavi)
Lower limbs	patella	pia ya mguu; iyitfu m'ivi
Lower limbs	lower leg	umurundi
Lower limbs	shin	umurundi
Lower limbs	calf	ifundo

Body parts	English	Kirundi
Lower limbs	ankle	urwambariro
Lower limbs	achilles' tendon	ikigango
Lower limbs	heel	igitsintsiri
Lower limbs	foot (feet)	ikirenge (ibirenge)
Lower limbs	big toe	ino rinini
Lower limbs	toe (toes)	ino (amano)
Lower limbs	toenail	urwara rw'ino

English	Kirundi
abdomen *The portion of the body bordered by the diaphragm and the pelvis.*	inda
abdominal girth *Waist circumference.*	amaraso ava ku'mutima, yamare ashike h'inyuma y'umuwiri
abdominocentesis *Puncturing of the abdominal wall for drainage purposes.*	Kuvoma amazi munda
abduct *To move a body part away from the body.*	kwigizayo igihimba c umubiri
aberrant *Different than normal.*	kitarico namba
abnormal, to be	kujujuta
ABO system *The system using human blood antigens to determine blood type.*	Imigwi y ' amaraso ABO
abortion (miscarriage) *Premature expulsion of the fetus from the uterus.*	ukuruhira ubusa
abortion, inevitable *Presence of cervical dilation or ruptured membranes in a pregnancy where the baby is not viable.*	Gukorora imbanyi,
above	hejuru
abrasion *Superficial skin injury.*	umuramu
abrupt *Suddenly or hastily.*	cihuta
abscess *A localized collection of pus.*	igihute
abscess, vulvar *Collection of pus and swelling of the vulva.*	ikihute cy'ikituba
absence of	igisibo
absolutely	rwose
abstain, to *To give up or to stop.*	gusiba
abuse, to (verbal abuse)	gushinyaguriza
accelerate *(To accelerate the healing process).*	kwongeza
access *Means of entry.*	ugushika
accessory *Complimentary or concomitant.*	y'inyuma; amongero
accident	icyago; icaduka; igisida
accommodation *A term used to describe the ability of the eye to adjust to various distances.*	icumbi
accomplish, to *Achieve.*	guheraheza
according to	kubwa
acephalous *A absence of a head.*	igihume
ache *A mild pain*	uburibwe
achieve, to *To complete something one was striving for.*	guheza
Achilles tendon *Also called calcaneal tendon; tendon with insertion at the gastrocnemius & soleus into the tuberosity of the calcaneus*	ikigango
acid *Substance with a pH less than 7.*	karu
acne *Inflamed or infected sebaceous glands.*	ikisigo
acoustic *Referring to the auditory system.*	umukenke w'ukumuwiriz' awarwaye

49

English	Kirundi
acquaint, to *To make someone familiar with something.*	kumenya
Acquired Immunodeficiency Syndrome (AIDS) *Presence of an AIDS defining illness or having a CD4 of less than 200/mm3.*	sida
acute *Abrupt onset* of disease.	indwara irenze urugero
Adam's apple *A prominence on the anterior neck caused by the thyroid cartilage of the larynx.*	akamirampeke
add, to *To count.*	kugereka
addiction *An abnormal dependency.*	kuromora
adenitis *The inflammation of a gland.*	ikinyawashi
adenopathy *Generally referring to a condition of the lymphatic glands.*	Isumbi
adequate *Sufficient.*	gikwiye
adherence *To stick to something figuratively or literally.*	kumata
adjacent, to be *To be in proximity to.*	kubangikana
adjust, to *To modify a plan.*	guhindura
adjustment *A modification of a plan.*	impinyanyuro
adjuvant *Term used to describe the medical treatment after initial therapy, as in adjuvant radiation therapy after initial chemotherapy.*	Umuti winyongera
admission (to hospital) *To be admitted.*	kwinjiza umuntu mu bitaro
adolescence	ubuyabaga
adult *Generally considered a person over 18 years old.*	umuntu akuze
adverse effect *In reference to medication use, it is an undesirable consequence of the drug.*	inkurikizi zimiti
advice *Recommendations regarding prudent further actions.*	inama
advise, to *To give counsel.*	guhanura
afebrile *Absence of fever.*	kudashuha (eg.he is afebrile: Ntashushe)
affect *The expression of emotions or feelings.*	gukorako
affinity *To have a natural liking for.*	ihuriro
after *The time following an event.*	inyuma
after-pains *The pain experienced after childbirth caused by uterine contractions.*	imisonga yo mugitereko
after-taste *The sensation of a prolonged savor following eating/ drinking.*	akanovera
afterbirth *The tissue expelled after the birth of a child that includes the placenta and allied membranes.*	ingovyi
again *Once more.*	ukundi
age *Length of life.(old age)*	ubukuru
aggression *Violent or hostile behavior.*	insondo
agitate, to *To cause a state of extreme emotional disturbance.*	kuzungagiza
agony, to be in *Anguish or torment.*	gusamba
agoraphobia *The fear of being in a large open space.*	Kutarinda
agreement *Accordance in opinion or feeling.*	igikumu
ague *A term used to describe recurrent fever and shivering typically associated with malaria.*	gutetemera
AIDS *Acquired Immunodeficiency Syndrome*	SIDA

English	Kirundi
AIDS, person living with	umuntu agendana umugera wa SIDA
air	impwemu
air hunger *The sensation of shortness of breath.*	kubura impemu
albino *A person who lacks pigment in the eyes, skin and hair.*	nyamwero
alcohol *Ethanol or ethyl alcohol.*	inzoga
alcoholism *An addiction to alcohol.*	kuborerwa
alert, to be *Being in a watchful, ready state.*	kuba maso
alexia *Inability to read due to a central brain lesion.*	kutamenya gusoma
algid *cold*	imbeho
allergy *An immune response by the body to a compound it is hypersensitive to.*	inyankane
alleviate, to	kugabanya
alopecia *The absence of hair in areas where it normally exists.*	ubuhanza
also *In addition.*	kandi
alteration *The process of change or modification.*	ihinduka
Alzheimer's disease *A dementia of unknown cause or pathogenesis.*	ubusazi
ambulance *A vehicle that carries the sick or injured.*	imodoka itwara abagwaye; ambilansi
ambulate, to *Relating to walking.*	kugenda
amenorrhea *The absence of menses.*	ubutinyanka
amentia *The absence of mental ability.*	kutagira ubwenge bukwiye
amnesia *The inability to remember past events.*	indwara y'urwiba
amniocentesis *Transabdominal aspiration of amniotic fluid.*	kuvoma amazi mugitereko
amnion *The membrane lining the placenta which produces the amniotic fluid.*	agasaho gahingura amazi yumwana
amniotic fluid *The fluid surrounding the fetus.*	uruziruzi
amount *The total or the aggregate.*	urugero
amputation *Typically referring to the surgical removal of a limb.*	uwugegeni
anal fistula *An opening in the skin that tracts to the anal canal thus causing some fecal material to leak from the opening in the skin.*	agakomere ko mugisusu
anal *Near or referring to the anus.*	mu gisusu
anal sphincter *Ring of striated muscle fibers surrounding the anus.*	amagara y'inyo
anal ulcer *An open wound near the anus.*	umuzimbwe
analgesia *The absence of pain.*	ukugabanya
analgesic *A medication used to remove pain.*	umuti ugabanya ububabare
analogous *To resemble or be similar to.*	gishusha
anastomosis *Surgical formation of a connection between two previously separate parts.*	gushona umubiri
anemia *Lower than normal red blood cell count.*	indrwara yo gukama amaraso
anencephaly *The congenital absence of the cranial vault and cerebral hemispheres.*	igihume
anesthesia *Loss of sensation.*	Gutimbsha
anesthetic *A chemical that produces anesthesia.*	umuti wo gutimbisha

English	Kirundi
aneurysm *A condition exhibited by the dilatation of the walls of an artery or vein to form a blood-filled sac.*	umudzi w'amaraso urarimvye
anger *A strong feeling of annoyance or hostility.*	uburake; ishavu
angina pectoris *Exercise induced myocardial ischemia.*	ibimirimiro
angioedema *Also called angioneurotic edema, it is caused by a histamine reaction. It can produce welts in mild cases but in severe cases can cause swelling of the lips and tongue.*	akasambangwiga
anguish *Significant mental or physical pain.*	iganya
anisomelia *Unequal size of arms or legs.*	kugira amagura n amaboko bitangana
ankle *The area of the ankle joint.*	ijisho ry'ikirenge; urwambariro
ankle edema or dependent edema *Extracellular fluid volume noted by swelling or pitting.*	kuvyimba amaguru
ankle joint *The articulation of the tibia/fibula and talus.*	urwambariro
ankle swelling *Enlargement of the ankle region with or without pitting.*	kuvyimba ijisho ryikirenge
anomia *Inability to name or recognize familiar objects.*	urwibagiza
anorchous *The absence of testicles.*	kutagira amavya
anorexia *The loss of appetite.*	ugutakaza akayabagu
anosmia *Lack of the sense of smell.*	kutahembera
anovulatory cycle *A menstrual cycle in which no ovum is released.*	kuja mukwegi umwigeme akabura urubuto rusohoka
anoxia *Reduced oxygen levels in body tissues.*	gukeha impemu mumubiri
antecubital fossa *The hollow at the bend of the elbow.*	umonga w'ukuwoko
antenatal *Refers to events before birth.*	imbere y amavuko
anterior *Toward the front.*	imbere
anthelmintic *An agent used to destroy worms.*	imiti yinzoka
anthrax *An infectious disease caused by Bacillus anthracis; there are cutaneous, inhalation and gastrointestinal syndromes.*	umugera w indwara y urukoma
anti-diarrheal *Medication used to treat diarrhea.*	imiti yo gucibwamo
anti-inflammatory *Medication used to reduce inflammation.*	imiti y ubushe bwumubiri
antibiotic *A medication that inhibits or kills microorganisms.*	umuti mponyamigera
antibody *A protein that combines with and counteracts foreign substances.*	umusoda womu mubiri
anticoagulant *Medication used to inhibit coagulation.*	imiti irwanya kuvura kwamaraso
anticonvulsant *Medication used to treat seizures.*	imiti y ibisahuzi
antidepressant *Medication used to treat depression.*	imiti yo kkuyinga
antidote *A medication that neutralizes a toxin.*	umuti uvura uburozi bwiyindi miti
antiemetic *A medication used to control nausea.*	umuti wo kudahwa
antimalarial *Medication used to treat malaria.*	umuti winyonko
antimigraine *Medication used to treat headaches.*	umuti wumutwe
antipruritic *Medication used to treat pruritus.*	umuti wuduhere two kurukoba
antipyretic *Medication used to treat fever.*	amuti wubushuhe
antitussive *Medication used to diminish a cough.*	umti winkorora
antivenin *An antitoxin formulated for various types of snake bites.*	umuti wubumara bwinzoka

English	Kirundi
anuria *The lack of urine excretion.*	kubura umukoyo
anus *The body opening distal to the rectum.*	inyo
anxiety *Nervousness or unease.*	amaganya
anxious *Experiencing nervousness or unease.*	kubuyabuya
aorta *The large artery originating at the left ventricle and going to the pelvis where it bifurcates.*	umuringoti utwara amaraso wo munda
aortic valve *The valve situated between the left ventricle and the aorta.*	udutemere two mu mitsi itwara amaraso
apart, to be *Separated by a distance.*	gushanyuka
apathy *Lack of interest in one's environment or indifference.*	igikonyo
apex *The highest point of something.*	agatwe
aphagia *The lack of eating.*	kutafungura
aphasia *Diminished ability to communicate via speech or writing.*	nyamuragi
aphonia *The loss of voice.*	kusarara
apnea *Absence of respiration.*	gukatika impemu
apoplexy *Extravasation of blood within an organ. For example, neonatal apoplexy is consistent with intracranial hemorrhage.*	ipasuka ry imiringoti itwara amaraso mu bwonko
appearance *The way someone looks or presents.*	ububoneke
appendectomy *Surgical excision of the appendix.*	kubagwa agasaho k'umusenyi k'urusogi
appendicitis *Inflammation of the appendix.*	ivyimba ry'agasaho k'umusenyi k'urusogi
appendix *An appendage of the cecum.*	agasaho k'umusenyi k'urusogi
appetite *A desire to eat.*	inambu
application *The forms one fills out to obtain a grant.*	umwete
applicator *A device used to apply a topical medication.*	akuma ko gusiga umuti kurukoba
appointment *A previously scheduled time to see a person.*	ihuriro
apprehensive *A fear that something unpleasant will happen.*	amakenga
approve, to *Accepting something as satisfactory.*	kwemera
approximate, to *To bring together, as in wound margins.*	kugera
approximately *Nearly but not completely.*	nka
aptitude *A natural talent for something.*	ingabirano
aptyalism *Diminished or absence of saliva.*	gukama amate
aqueous humor *The fluid between the cornea and lens, anterior to the globe.*	igihimba cijisho
arachnodactyly *A condition exhibited by abnormally long and slender fingers.*	intoke ndende
argue, to *To debate or reason. (quarrel)*	guharira
arm *One of two upper extremities. (arms)*	ukuboko (amaboko)
arm, upper	ikizigira
arm, left	ukuboko kw'ibubamfu
arm, right	ukuboko kw'iburyo
armpit *A common term for axilla.*	ukwaha
around, to be *To be on every side of.*	gukikira
arrhythmia *An abnormal heart rhythm.*	isimbagurika ry umutima

English	Kirundi
arteriosclerosis *Hardening and thickening of arterial walls.*	ivyimba ry imiringoti itwara amaraso
arteritis *Inflammation of an artery.*	ubushe bwimitsi itwara amaraso
artery *Vessel that carries oxygenated blood from the heart to the periphery.*	umutsi uvana amaraso mu mutima
arthritis *Joint inflammation.*	indwara ifata amahuriro y'amagufwa
artificial *Not natural produced.*	c'ighimbano
ascaricide *Agent that destroys ascaris.*	inganga
ascaris *A nematode from genus intestinal lumbricoid parasite, also called round worm.*	inzoka yo munda
ascertain, to *Synonym of "to determine".*	kugena
ascites *Serous fluid in the abdominal cavity.*	urusina
asepsis *Lack of infection.*	umubiri usaneza
asleep *To be in a dormant or inactive state.*	itiro
aspermia *Absence of sperm.*	gukama intanga
asphyxia *A condition exhibited by a lack of oxygen and subsequent loss of consciousness or death.*	ukubura impwemu
aspiration biopsy *Removal of fluid from a cavity for pathologic analysis.*	kuvoma amazi mumubiri yo kuja gupima
assessment *An medical evaluation.*	isuzuma
assistance *The act of helping.*	kugomorera
asthenia *Diminished strength and energy.*	kubura inguvu
asthma *An inflammatory disease of the lungs noteworthy because of reversible airway obstruction.*	asima
asymmetry *Lack of symmetry.*	bidatumberanye
asymptomatic *The absence of symptoms.*	atakimenyetso cindwara
at random *Occurring by chance alone.*	kwa tombora
ataxia *Lack of muscular coordination.*	kudatemebreza ibihimba vyumubiri neza
athetosis *An involuntary symptom exhibited by continuous slow, writhing movements, mostly in the hands.*	kutayobora ukuboko
athlete's foot *Common term for tinea pedis.*	indwara yo mu kirenge
atrium *Referring to a chamber used as an entrance, as in the entrance to the heart.*	agasaho ko mumutima
atrophy *A diminution in the size of a part.*	ubupfunya
atrophy of a paralyzed extremity	kumugaza
atypical *Not usual.*	kitameze nk'ibindi
audiologist *A clinician specializing in disorders of the ear.*	muganga w'amatwi
auditory agnosia *Caused by a temporal lobe lesion, it is characterized by inability to recognize sounds as words.*	indwara yo kutumva neza
auditory canal, external *Also called the external acoustic meatus; it leads from the auricle to the tympanic membrane.*	iyomviro
auricle *The external portion of the ear.*	ugutwi
auricular nerve *Nerve supplying the ear.*	umudzi w'amatwi
auscultate, to *The act of listening to sounds emanating from the body.*	gusuzuma

English	Kirundi
autopsy *Examination of a body post-mortem in an attempt to determine cause of death.*	ugusuzuma umuvyimba
availability *A person or thing that is available.*	ukuboneka
available *Attainable, obtainable.*	kuboneka
avoidable *That which can be stopped or inhibited.*	gishobora kwirindwa
awakening *The state of being conscious.*	kugaba, gukanura
away from *Separated from.*	kure
axilla *The hollow beneath the arm.*	ukwaha; ubwakwaka
baby *A newborn.(babies)*	umwana (abana)
baby-scale *A device used to weigh an infant.*	umunzane upima inzoya
back *The back of a person.*	umugongo
backbone *Spine.*	urutirigongo
back pain *Discomfort on the dorsal surface of the torso.*	umugongo (kurwara)
bacteria *Plural for any organism of the order Eubacteriales.*	umugera
balanitis *Inflammation of the glans of the penis.*	indwara yo mu nzanyi
balm *A topical medical preparation.*	amafata y'ukwisiga
bandage *A strip of gauze used to immobilize or support.*	ugutenga
bandage tied to a circumcised penis	ipansuma yo ku nzanyi
basin *A small bowl used for washing.*	ikarabo
basophil *A polymorphonuclear granulocyte.*	ubwoko bwabasoda bumubiri
bathing *To wash oneself.*	umwuhagiro
bear, to *To endure or resist.*	kwihangana
bear, to *To give birth to a child.*	guhonoka
bearing down *As in during labor.*	guhamangira
beat *As in heart beat.*	gutera indihaguzi
bed rest *A medical order requiring one to stay in bed.*	kuruhuka mugitanda bisabwe na muganga
bedbug Cimex lectularius. *A small insect that is parasitic and hides in clothing or bedding.*	igihere
bedpan *A metal or plastic vestibule one sits on while in bed to defecate.*	icombo abagwaye bitumamwo
bedridden *Term used to indicate one is so ill they cannot get out of bed.*	kuvundira mu gitanda
bed *A mattress resting on a frame.*	uburiri
beer *A form of fermented alcohol. (banana beer)*	inzoga (urwarwa)
bee sting *A piercing from a bee.*	uruboyi
beforehand *In advance or previously.*	imbere
behavior disorder *An abnormal mental state.*	indwara yo kwifata nabi
belch, to *Eructation.*	gutura amangati
Bell's palsy *Unilateral facial paralysis related to dysfunction of the seventh cranial nerve.*	kumugara igice co mumaso bivuye kukutetera kw umutsi nsoza bwenge ugira indwi
below *Under.*	hepfo
benign *Not harmful. (benign condition)*	ata inabi (indwara itagira uwubi)
bereaved, to be *The sorrow one feels with the loss of a loved one.*	kuvubga

English	Kirundi
best *Optimal or ideal.*	iza
beyond, to go *To go further.*	kurenga
biased *Prejudiced.*	guhengama
bilateral *Referring to both sides.*	impande zose
bile *An alkaline fluid secreted by the liver to aid digestion.*	indurwe
bile ducts *The structures that are conduits for passage of bile from the liver and gallbladder to the duodenum.*	imiringoti y indugu
Bilharzia *Historical name of a genus of flukes or nematodes now known as Schistosoma.*	Birariziose
bill *A financial statement that indicates how much one owes.*	ifagitire
biology *The study of living organisms.*	icigwa c'ibinyabuzima
birth *The process of bearing offspring from the uterus.*	ivuka
birth control *Any method of limiting contraception.*	ukuvyara ku rugero
birth defect *A congenital anomaly.*	ubumuga bw'ubuvukano
birthmark *A benign brown or red patch one is born with.*	ikibibi
bistoury; scalpel *A surgical knife.*	Imbugita yo kwa muganga
bitter (taste) *Having a harsh, unpleasant taste.*	kururirwa
black *Referring to the color, as in the color of coal.*	umufyiri
black stools *Common term for melena.*	kwituma amaraso yirabura
blackout *Common term for loss of consciousness.*	ukuraba
blackwater fever *A term used to describe the fever associated with malaria when the urine is reddish-black.*	indwara y ubushuhe n umukozo utukura bivuye ku inyonko
bladder, urinary *Vestibule for urine prior to being expelled via the urethra.*	uruhago
bleed, to *Loss of blood.*	kuva amaraso
blemish *A small mark on one's skin.*	agatosi
blepharitis *Inflammation of the eyelids.*	indwara y amaso
blepharospasm *A spasm of the orbicularis oculi muscle that causes closure of the eyelid.*	indwara yo gusinzira ijisho rimwe
blind person *Person with absence of sight.*	impumyi
blind, to be *To have an absence of visual perception.*	guhuma
blink, to *To open and close the eyelid rapidly.*	guhumaguza
blister *Common term for bulla.*	ibavu
bloated *Sensation of having an abnormally large amount of air in the viscera.*	kubondoka
blood *Plasma containing erythrocytes, leukocytes and platelets.*	amaraso
blood alcohol level *A quantitative measurement of the amount of alcohol in the blood.*	ugupima urugero rwinzoga mu maraso
blood cells *A common term that does not differentiate between erythrocyte or leukocyte.*	abasoda bumubiri
blood clot *A mass of coagulated blood.*	umugoma
blood grouping *Testing blood to determine which type should be used for transfusion.*	umurwi wamaraso
blood pressure *Written as the measurement in mmHg at the time of systole of the left ventricle over the time of diastole.*	umurindi w'amaraso
blood stream *(blood vessel) Common term or the arterial or venous systems.*	umutsi
blood type *Determined and listed in the ABO system.*	umurwi w'amaraso

blood-letting *The removal of blood from a patient with the thought it would cure or prevent disease.*   kurumika

blow one's nose, to   kwimyira

blue *A color between green and violet.*   ubururu

blunt *Having a flat or rounded end.*   gifushe

blurred vision *Low visual acuity. (fuzzy vision)*   kuzimangana

blurt out, to *To speak without considering the repercussions.*   gufudika

blush, to *To have an increased volume of blood flow to one's face causing a red tint to the skin.*   gutukura

body surface area *Dubois formula is: (weight in kilograms)to the 0.425th power x (height in centimeters) to the 0.725th power x 0.007184.*   igipimo cibiro nukwo umuntu angana

body *The physical structure of a person.*   umubiri

body weight *Relative mass as measured in kilograms or pounds.*   ibiro vy umubiri

boil *Small abscess or furuncle.*   igihute

bone *Skeletal tissue formed by osteoblasts.*   igufa

bone marrow *The soft material filling the cavity of bones.*   umusokoro

born, to be *Being present as a result of birth.*   kuvuka

bottle *A container used for the storage of liquids.*   icupa

bow-legged *Synonym for genu varum.*   amaguru y'imbango

brace *A splint.*   udukore sho babohesha uwavunitse

brace, to *Application of a splint.*   guhimbura

brachial plexus *A cluster of nerves coming off the last four cervical and first thoracic spinal nerves form the nerve supply the the chest and arms.*   ihuriro ry imitsi mu kuboko

bradycardia *Lower than normal cardiac rate measured in beats per minute.*   umutima utera bukebuke

brain *A common term for cerebrum.*   ubgonko; ubwonko

brain death *Cessation of cerebral functioning.*   ugupfa kw ubwonko

brain stem *An organ that consists of the medulla oblongata, pons and midbrain. (base of the brain)*   agakomokomo

break, to (as in bone) *A common term for a fracture in a bone.*   kuvuna

breast *Mammary tissue including the areola.*   ibere

breast abscess *Pus collection in the breast.*   ikisebe cy'ikiwere

breast feeding *The process of giving milk to a baby via the nipple.*   kwonsa

breast milk   amaberebere

breath *One respiration.*   impwemu

breath sounds *The noise heard upon auscultation with a stethoscope.*   kwumva umuntu ariko arahema

breath test (for alcohol) *A check of alcohol level by testing exhaled air.*   gupima inzoga mumpwemu

breathe, to *The act of respiration.*   guhema; guhumeka

breathing   ugusohora impwemu

breathing in   ukwinjiza impwemu

breech birth *Delivery with the feet or buttocks coming first.*   kuvyaza umwana yicaye

English	Kirundi
breech presentation *Position of the feet or buttocks near the cervix.*	umwana yicaye
bright *Giving out a lot of light.*	umutari
bring, to *To carry or transport something.*	kuzana
brisk *Rapid or fast.*	in'ingoga
broken (arm) *Fracture of the arm.*	imvune ukuboko
bronchiole *A small branch that a bronchus divides into.*	uduce twamahaha
bronchitis *Inflammation of the mucous membranes of the bronchioles that causes bronchospasm and cough.*	indwara yuduce twamahaha
bronchus *The major air channels that bifurcate from the distal trachea.*	agahogohogo kaja mu mahaha
brow presentation *The term used to describe which part of the body (forehead) is being delivered first in childbirth.*	kuvuka umwana atanguje umutwe
brown *Coffee-colored.*	igihogo
bruise, to *Common term for to cause ecchymosis.*	guharura umubiri
brush teeth, to *Use of a toothbrush to clean the teeth.*	kwinyugunura indobo
bubo *An inflamed, swollen lymph node in the axilla or inguinal region.*	ikivimbe
bubonic plague *A form of plague exhibited by the formation of buboes.*	gahembe
buccal *Referring to the cheek.*	itama
bug *Insect.*	agasimba
bulge, to *Formation of a protuberance on a flat surface.*	kudundura
bulimia *Chronic condition characterized by secretive eating of large quantities of food followed by self-induced vomiting.*	uwuryi, inzara nyinshi
burn *An injury caused by exposure to heat.*	ubushe
burst, to *To rupture.*	kwaturura
buttocks (buttock) *The bilateral region covering the gluteal muscles.*	amatako (itako)
cachexia *Generalized weakness and severe wasting.*	kunamba cane
cadaver *A dead body.*	umuvyimba
calcaneus *Commonly called the heel bone.*	igitsintsiri
calcium *A chemical element that is an essential component in teeth and bone.*	ikarisiyumu
calculus *A stone of minerals that can lead to the blockage of the bile duct or ureters.*	akabuye ko mu ndugu
calf *Muscles of the posterior portion of the lower leg.*	intege
calf, soreness or pain in the	ikicyaganuzi
callosity *Callus; thickened hardened skin.*	ibavu
cancel, to *To stop or revoke.*	gufata
cancer; carcinoma *A disease of uncontrolled abnormal cell growth.*	kanseri
candle *A cylindrical piece of wax with a central wick.*	ishashara
cane *Device used to aid walking (walking stick).*	inkoni yo kwishimikiza
canine teeth *Located between the incisors and premolars.*	ibgena
canker sore *An ulceration, usually of the mouth or lips.*	ibisebe biterwa n'isuna
capillary *A vessel that connects arterioles to venules.*	udutsi nsanganya maraso
capsule *Medication in the form of a capsule.*	ikinini

English	Kirundi
caput *The head.*	umutwe
carbon monoxide poisoning *This tasteless, odorless gas causes constitutional symptoms but can lead to death upon inhalation.*	umwuka wubumara
cardiac *Referring to the heart.*	y'umutima
cardiac arrest *Cessation of function of the heart.*	ihagarara ry'umutima
cardiopulmonary resuscitation *Use of artificial means to support respiration and circulation.*	kuvura indembe y indwara y umutima n amahaha
cardiovascular *Referring to the heart or circulatory system.*	umutima n imitsi yamaraso
caregiver *A person who provides care to another.*	umurwaza
caries *Referring to decay or death of a tooth.*	ukubora kw'amenyo
carotid *Referring to the large artery on each side of the neck.*	munini uzana amaras mu'mutwe
carpopedal spasm *A spasm of the carpus and the foot.*	ipfunywa ry imitsi yo kukirenge
cartilage *Firm, relatively non-vascular connective tissue.*	igufa ry'igisigati
cast; plaster cast *Use of plaster of paris to immobilize an extremity.*	isima bashira ku mvune
castrate, to *Excision of the gonads.*	gukona
casualty *A person who is killed or seriously injured.*	uwagize
cataract *An opacity of an eye lens or the capsule.*	umurazi
catarrh *Inflammation of a mucous membrane.*	indwara y amaso
catch a cold *To come down with a viral upper respiratory tract infection.*	agaherera
catheter *A flexible tube inserted into the body.*	urushinge rwa parasitike rwo gucishamwo umuti
caudal *Referring to a cauda.*	kijanye n'umurizo
cavity *Pouch or chamber.*	akanogo
cecum *The first portion of the large intestine.*	umwinizirano
center *A point equidistant from all sides.*	hagati
central nervous system (CNS) *The brain and spinal cord.*	ubwonko n uruti rw umugongo
cephalic *Towards the head.*	kijanye n'umutwe
cerebellum *The part of the brain in the posterior portion of the skull that controls muscle coordination and movement.*	agakomokomo
cerebrospinal fluid (CSF) *The fluid between the pia mater and arachnoid membrane.*	amazi yo muruti rw umugongo
cerebrovascular accident (stroke) *A decrease in level of consciousness and paralysis caused by a cerebrovascular thrombosis, hemorrhage or vasospasm.*	n'indwara bukumbi y'ubwonko
cerumen impaction, to clean out *Cleansing of external ear canal because it is full of wax resulting in hearing loss.*	gukurugutura
cerumen *Waxy substance found normally in the external ear canals.*	ubukurugutwi
cervix uteri *The narrow end of the uterus.*	ubwinjiriro bw'igitereko
cesarean section *Incision of the abdominal and uterine walls in order to deliver a fetus when natural delivery is not possible.*	gusatura mu nda mu kukuvyaza
chalazion *A chronic inflammatory granuloma of a meibomian gland; also called meibomian cyst.*	utuherehere
chancre *The initial ulcer that is seen with primary syphilis.*	mburugu
check for, to	guhinyuza

59

English	Kirundi
cheek *Lateral facial tissue.*	itama
cheekbone	agasendabageni
chemotherapy *Use of medication (chemical agents) in the treatment of disease. This term is commonly used to refer to the treatment of cancer patients with medication.*	kuvuza imiti, canecane ku ndwara ya kanseri
chest *Thorax.*	igikiriza
chew, to *Masticate.*	gutapfuna
chicken pox, varicella *A viral disease characterized by extremely pruritus blisters over the entire body.*	agasama
chigger *A parasitic mite of the genus Trombicula.*	indwara y inzoka
child *A person aged 1 to 8 years old. (male, female)*	umugimbi
childbirth *Parturition; the process of labor and delivery of an infant.*	igise
childhood *The time between infancy and puberty.*	ubgana
chills *Sensation of coldness.*	agashitsi
chin *Mentum; the anterior projection of the lower jaw.*	urusagusagu; urusakanwa
choose, to *To make an election or decision.*	gutora
choke *To retch, cough or fight for breath.*	kuniga
cholecystectomy *Surgical excision of the gallbladder.*	kubaga indugu
cholecystitis *Inflammation of the gallbladder.*	indwara y indugu
cholera *An infectious disease exhibited by vomiting and diarrhea and caused by Vibrio cholerae.*	korera
cholesterol *A compound or its derivatives are found in cell membranes and precursors to hormones but high levels can cause atherosclerosis.*	amavuta yo mu mubiri
chronic *When referring to an illness, it means recurring or persistent.*	kidadera
cicatrix (scar) *New tissue in a healed wound.*	ururasago
cilia *The hairs growing on the eyelid or a motile extension of a cell surface.*	ingohe
circadian *Referring to a 24 hour period.*	igihe c amasaha 24
circumcise, to *To surgically excise the foreskin.*	kugenyera
circumcision *The surgical excision of foreskin.*	ugusiramura
circumference *The distance around an object or part.*	inkikuro
cirrhosis *A liver disease characterized by destruction of liver cells and increased connective tissue.*	urusina
clavicle *A bone that articulates with the sternum and scapula.*	umugororo
clear one's throat, to *To cough lightly in attempt to speak more clearly.*	gukorora imbere yo kuvuga utomora
clear *Transparent.*	kubonerana
clearance *The process of removing something.*	gukuraho
cleavage *A sharp division or demarcation.*	igabanganya
cleft lip *A congenital abnormal opening of the lip.*	umunwa mubi
clinic *A building where patients are evaluated.*	ivuriro
clitoris *A small erectile body in the anterosuperior aspect of the vulva.*	ikinena; akusino
close, to	gufunga
clot *A thrombus or embolus.*	urubu

English	Kirundi
cluster headache *A unilateral, severe, recurrent headache.*	kumeneka umutwe uruhande rumwe
coagulate, to *The formation of a clot.*	gufatana
coccyx *The small bone formed by the natural fusion of rudimentary vertebrae.*	igufa ry'ikiwuno
cochlea *The essential organ of hearing which is in a spiral form.*	igihimba co mugutwi
cockroach *A beetle-like insect with long legs and antennae.*	inyenzi
cognition *The process of acquiring thought or understanding.*	ubumenyi
coitus *Sexual intercourse between members of the opposite sex.*	uguhuza ibitsina
cold *Having a sense of being cold.*	-bisi
cold sore *A perioral blister caused by herpes simplex.*	amahere y'inyonko
cold *Viral upper respiratory tract infection.(cold in head)*	agahehera (agahiri)
colectomy *Surgical removal of part of the colon.*	kubaga amara
colic *Acute abdominal pain.*	ikisigo
colitis *Inflammation of the colon.*	indwara y amara
collapse *To have a physical or mental breakdown.*	guhenuka
collarbone *Common term for the clavicle.*	umugororo
colon *The portion of the large intestine that goes from the cecum to the rectum.*	umurungoro
color blindness *The inability to distinguish colors.*	indwara yo kudatandukanya amabara
colostrum *The fluid secreted by the mammary glands a few days around parturition.*	umuhondo
coma *A state of unconsciousness.*	ukuraba
comment *A remark providing an opinion.*	ugushima kw'umwigisha
common, to be *That which is usual.*	kuba ibisanzwe
compatible *To coexist without problems.*	bijanye
compendium *A concise summary about a subject.*	incamake
complaint *Grievance.*	umwidodombo
compliance *The act of going along with a plan.*	ukujana
comply, to *Adhere to.*	kwoma
compound *A substance formed by covalent union of two or more atoms.*	urucange
comprehend, to *To understand.*	gutahura
concentric *Referring to circles or arcs that share the same center.*	bifise umukondo umwe
conception *The act of an egg being fertilized by sperm.*	gusama inda
concussion *Head trauma resulting in temporary loss of consciousness.*	kugira isangaya ryo mumutwe
condom *A covering for the penis or the vagina (female condom) used during sexual intercourse that is meant to reduce the chance of pregnancy or infection.*	agakingirizo; udufuko
confabulation *The fabrication of experiences to compensate for memory loss.*	ivyaremetanijwe
confidence *Self-assurance.*	icizigiro
confinement *As in confined to bed.*	ubgiba
conflict *Dispute or disagreement.*	gutata
confusion *Disorientation.*	umuvurngano

61

English	Kirundi
congenital defect *A disease or anomaly present from birth.*	ikigaga
congenital syphilis *Passed to the child in utero, the child may have failure to thrive, fever and a flattened bridge of the nose.*	agashangara (c'ikivukano)
congestive heart failure *A diminished cardiac output leading to passive engorgement.*	uguhagarara umutima
conjunctiva *The membrane that lines the eyelid.*	igice c ijisho
conjunctivitis *Inflammation of the conjunctiva.*	uburire
conscious *Being award and being able to respond to one's surroundings.*	kuba maso
consistent *Compatible with something or congruous with.*	gihuye na
constipation *A condition exhibited by difficulty in having a bowel movement due to hard stools.*	igisigo
constriction *Circumferential tightening*	agahato
contact *The touching of two bodies or a person who has been exposed to a contagious disease.*	ugukora ku
contagious, to be *Description of a disease that can be spread by direct or indirect contact.*	kwandukira
contaminate, to *To make impure by exposing to an polluted agent.*	gutobeka
content *What something is made up of.*	ibirimwo
contraceptive *A device or medication used to prevent pregnancy.*	uburyo bwo kuvyara kurugero
contraceptives, oral *A medication taken by mouth by a woman to prevent pregnancy.*	ibinini vyo kumira
contractions *Abdominal muscle contractions during the last weeks of pregnancy.*	nk'ibise
contradictory *Two elements that are inconsistent.*	gihushanye
contradication *A situation in which two elements are inconsistent.*	uguhushanya
convenient *Opportune or well-timed.*	gikwiriye
convulsions *An involuntary series of tonic and clonic movements.*	ukudadarara kw'imitsi
cool *Chilly or cold.*	ugufuta
cope, to *To deal with a difficult situation.*	kwimenya
cord compression *Pressure being applied to the spinal cord.*	ifyondekara ry imitsi yuruti rwumugongo
cornea *The transparent segment located at the anterior part of the eye.*	igice kibonerana co mujisho
cornea prolapse *Protrusion of the cornea from injury.*	idzjicyo riramenese
corneal transplant *Surgical replacement of a cornea with a donor cornea.*	kubaga bagasubiriza igice kibonerana co mujisho

English	Kirundi
corpulence *Fatness.*	ubuvyibuhe
coryza *An acute condition exhibited by copious nasal discharge.*	ikiseru
cost *The fee or penalty.*	igiciro
cotton wool *Raw cotton.*	ipampa
cough *Forceful expulsion of air from the lungs.*	inkorora
coughing fit *An episode of prolonged, forceful coughing.*	agahehera
cough, to	gukorora
count, to *To determine a number.*	guharura
cow's milk	amata
crab louse *Phthirus pubis is formal name for a louse that infests pubic hair and causes intense itching.*	inda
cramp *A painful contraction of muscles.*	imbwa
crave,to *An unusually strong urge for something.*	gukenera birengeye urugero
cripple *A person with a physical disability; not used in polite society.*	ikimuga
crisis *A turning point in the treatment of a disease.*	amagume
croup *An acute laryngeal condition that is accompanied by a hoarse, barking cough.*	ikisheshwe
crust *Dried serous exudate covering a wound.*	uwukarabe
crutches *Long metal or wooden sticks used for support while walking.*	amabekire
CSF *Abbreviation for cerebrospinal fluid.*	Amazi yo muruti rwumugongo
cumulative effect *A consequence of successive additions.*	kigenda ciyongera
cuneiform *The three bones between the navicular bone and the metatarsals.*	Igufa rzo mu gikonjo
curative *A remedy capable of healing completely.*	Umuti Ukiza
cure *A remedy for a medical illness.*	umuti
curettage *Removal of tissues from a cavity.*	Gukoropa mu bihimba vyirondoka
curette *The instrument used during a curettage.*	Icuma bakoresha mu gukoropa mumubiri
current *Flow or stream.*	umukuba
currently *Presently.*	kiboneka cane
cushion *A pillow or stuffed pad used to sit on.*	umusego
cut *An incision.*	uruguma
cuticle *The dead skin at the base of the toenail or fingernail, also called the eponychium.*	Umubiri woboze
cyanosis *Bluish discoloration of the skin and mucous membranes.*	kwirabura umubiri bivuye mu kubura impwemu mu mubiri

63

English	Kirundi
cyclical vomiting *Periods of recurrent vomiting with no apparent pathologic cause and the person has a normal state of health between the episodes.*	Kudahwa umwanya wose
cynocephaly *Craniostenosis in which the cranium slopes back from the orbits.*	inguge
cystic fibrosis *A congenital disorder exhibited by abnormal thick mucous which leads to problems in the intestines, pancreas and lungs.*	Indwaraa yo munda ifata amara, urwagasha, n amahaha
cystitis *Inflammation of the urinary bladder.*	Indwara yo mukayiba kinda
dacryocystitis *Inflammation of a lacrimal sac.*	Indwara zuturingoti dutwara amosozi
dandruff *Dead skin found in the hair.*	indwara y'uburima
date of admission *Beginning date of hospitalization.*	Itariki yo kwinjira mubitaro
date of birth	isabukuru y'amavuka
daughter	umukobga
dead, to be *Deceased. (dead person)*	gupfa
deadline *Cutoff date.*	igihe ntarengwa
deaf *Absence of the sense of hearing. (deaf person)*	igipfamatwi
deaf-mute *Inability to hear or speak.*	ikiragi
deafness *Having impaired hearing.*	ubupfamatwi
death *The action of dying.*	urupfu
debility *Physical weakness.*	ubugugu
debridement *Trimming the dead tissue adjacent to a wound.*	gukurako ikintu
decade *Ten years.*	ikiringo c'imyaka cumi
decapitate, to *The physical separation of the head from the body.*	guca umutwe
deciduous teeth,to get one's first or *The first teeth.*	kwera
decline *As in a decrease in status or health.*	gutakaze
decrease *Becoming smaller or fewer.*	gukama
decubitus *Laying flat in bed or dorsal decubitus. (lateral decubitus is flat and on one's side)*	Kuryama ugaramye
decubitus ulcer *A wound caused by laying in one position for too long; also referred to as a pressure ulcer.*	kubora umubiri (bivuye mukumara igihe kirekire uryamye)
deep *Having significant depth.*	-rere
deep vein thrombosis (DVT) *A blood clot that forms within a vein, typically in the lower extremities.*	Indwara y imitsi
deer tick *Ixodes scapularis.*	igitangu (ifumberi)
defecate *To discharge feces from the rectum.*	kunya
defect, speech *A shortcoming or imperfection in speech*	ubureve
deficiency *Insufficiency or deficit.*	ubukene
deformity *A malformation or imperfection.*	ubumuga
deglutition *The process of swallowing.*	kumira
dehydration *The status of having a decrease in total body water.*	ugukama amazi
delirium;to be delirious *An acute mental state exhibited by altered thought processes and restlessness.*	ukudedemda (kudedemba)

English	Kirundi
delirium tremens *A condition seen when alcohol is withdrawn which is exhibited by restlessness, hallucinations and tremors.*	indwara yo mumutwe iterwa no guhagarika inzoga bukwi na bukwi
deliver,to (a child) *The process of giving birth. (forceps delivery)*	kuvyara
delusion *A belief that is contradictory to rational thought.*	indwara yo mumutwe ituma umuntu yemeza ibitarivyo
demarcation *Having a fixed boundary.*	urubibe
dementia *A chronic brain disorder exhibited by memory loss, personality changes and faulty reasoning.*	ubusazi
dengue *A mosquito-borne viral disease exhibited by fever and joint pain.*	Indwara ya dengue
density *The denseness of an object.*	ubureme
dental *Referring to teeth.*	kijanye n'amenyo
dental caries *Decay of teeth.*	ibungwe ry'iryinyo
dentist *A professional capable of treating diseases of the teeth and gums.*	umuganga w'amenyo
dentures *A frame that holds artificial teeth.*	amenyo y'amaterano
deny, to *To reject or repudiate.*	guhakana
depo-vera injection *A birth control medication injected every three months.*	inshinge bita "depo-vera injections"
depression *A medical condition exhibited by profound despondency.*	akabonge
deprivation *The lack of a necessity.*	ukwima
dermatitis *Non-specific inflammation of the skin.*	indrwara y'ibubura ry'urukoba
dermis *The "true skin" that lies beneath the epidermis.*	uruhu
descending *Moving toward the inferior portion.*	kumanuka
desiccation *The act of drying up.*	gukamya
despite *Notwithstanding.*	n'ubwo
desquamation *The shedding of scales of any body surface.*	kwiyawira icyubu
deterioration *Worsening in one's medical condition.*	guseruka
detrimental *Harmful.*	kitera ingaruka mbi
deviation *Away from the norm.*	ihusha
diabetes mellitus *A disease exhibited by a deficiency of the pancreatic hormone insulin.*	indwara y'igisukari
diaphoretic *Exhibited by profuse perspiration.*	kubira icuya cane
diaphragm *The muscular separation between the thoracic and abdominal cavities.*	Inyama itandukanya amaha no munda
diarrhea *Increase in frequency and a loose consistency of the stools.*	agahitwe
diarrhea, to have *(verb) The act of having diarrhea.*	guhitwa
die, to *To stop living, to expire.*	gupfa
diet *The kinds of food a person eats.*	ingaburo
dietician *Clinician specializing in the treatment of nutrition related disorders.*	ujejwe kuraba ko abantu bafungura neza
differential diagnosis *A list of possible alternative diagnoses for a patient who is ill.*	Iyindi ndwara yishoboka
digestion *The process of enzymatic breakdown of food in the alimentary canal.*	isya ry'imfungurwa mu nda

English	Kirundi
digit *Finger.*	urutoke
dilatation *The process of becoming wider or larger.*	igaruka
dilator *An instrument that dilates.*	Icaguzo
dilution *The process of making a weaker solution.*	ifungura
diphtheria *A contagious bacterial disease characterized by a grey membrane on the pharynx along with respiratory or cutaneous symptoms; caused by Corynebacterium diphtheriae.*	diphtheria (ikirato)
diplegia *The paralysis of both arms or both legs.*	kumugara igice c umubiri
diplopia *Double vision.*	ukubona (kubiri)
dipsomania *Compulsion to drink alcoholic beverages.*	Kuboregwa
dirty *Unclean.*	ubucafu
disability *Decreased or impaired mental or physical ability.*	ubumuga
disappearance *An instance of something/someone gone missing.*	umushiro
disarticulation *Amputation through the joint.*	kucyira icyungiro
discharge,hospital *The release of a patient from the hospital.*	ugusohora umurwayi mu bitaro
discharge, ear *Otic secretions.*	ukuva amashira (ugutwi)
discharge, nasal *Nasal secretions.*	ikisere
discharge, postpartum vaginal *The secretions noted after delivery.*	Ibirashi
discharge, abnormal vaginal *Purulent vaginal secretions.*	ukuva amashira (igituba)
discomfort *A feeling of physical or mental unease.*	ububabare
discrete *Separate and distinct.*	kinyegeye
disease *Malady or disorder.*	indwara
disease outcome *The response obtained from treatment.*	iherezo ryo kuvugra
disequilibrium *The absence of stability.*	ihungabana
disinfectant *A substance that kills bacteria.*	umuti uhonya imigera
dislocation *The displacement of a bone when referring to an articulation. (sprain, dislocate, startle)*	gutandukana mu ngingo
dislocation, shoulder *Separation of the humerus from the scapula at the glenohumeral joint.*	kuvunika ku rutugu
disorder *Impairment.*	ingorane zo mu mubiri
disorientation *Mental confusion.*	uguta umutwe
displacement *Movement from normal position.*	isubirizwa
disrobe, to *To remove clothing.*	kwambura
dissemination *To be spread or dispersed widely.*	ikwiragizwa
distal *Situated away from the center of the body.*	Kwiherezo
distension *Swollen.*	ubutumbi
distribution *The manner in which something is shared or spread out.*	ugutanga
diuresis *Increased excretion of urine.*	Isohoka ry umukoyo
diuretic *Medication which causes an increased excretion of urine.*	kijanye no gutakaza amazi mu mubiri kubera ugusoba cane
dizziness,to have *Sensation of losing one's balance.*	kuzererwa
dorsal *Referring to the back or back surface.*	kijanye 'umugongo
dorsalis pedis pulse *Pulse on dorsum of the foot.*	itera ryimitsi y amaraso yo kukirenge

English	Kirundi
dosage *The amount and frequency a medication is given.*	ugutanga umuti
dosing interval *The number of times per unit a medication is given.*	Ugupima umuti
double *Twice the size, quantity or strength.*	kabiri
douche *Cleansing of a canal; unless otherwise specified it refers to cleansing of the vaginal canal.*	kwoza igisabo
down *In a lower position.*	hepfo
drastic *Having significant effect.*	gikabije
dream *The thoughts or images occurring during sleep.*	inzozi
dressing, to change a *To place a new dressing on a wound.*	guhindura ipansoma
dress,to *To apply gauze to a wound.*	gusomora
dribble, to *To slowly, drip-by-drip, release urine for example.*	dukeya twa inkari
drill *Cylindrical metal tool uses for creating a hole in bone in surgery.*	igitobozi
drink, to *To imbibe.*	kunywa
drinking water *Water clean enough to ingest orally.*	amazi
drop *A single bit of fluid as in a drop seen while giving IV fluids.*	intonyanga
drop by drop *Expression meaning little by little.*	akamakama
drops per minute *Refers to iv fluid rate.*	amama akoroka kumunota
drown,to *The process of dying from submerging in and inhaling water.*	gusoma nturi
drowsiness *Sleepiness.*	ugutura ingiga
drug *A medication, sometimes with negative connotation.*	ibyobezabwenge
drug dependence *Addiction to a substance.*	kuba umuja ibyobezabwenge
drug reaction *Typically refers to an adverse effect of medication.*	impinduka yumuti
drunk,to be *Inebriated.*	kuborerwa
dry *Absence of moisture.*	cumye
dry cough *A cough without sputum production.*	Inkorora yagahehera
dual diagnosis *Term used to describe the presence of alcohol/ drug addiction associated with a psychiatric diagnosis such as depression.*	Indwara yo mumutwe ivuye mu kuborerwa canke kufata imiti myinshi
duodenum *The portion of the small bowel between the stomach and jejunum.*	amara
duplication *The process of duplicating something.*	ukugwiza amakopi
dura mater *The outermost covering of the brain and spinal cord.*	Igice cubwonko
dust *Dry earthen particles found on the ground and surfaces.*	inkungugu
dwarf *Abnormally small person.*	igikuri
dysarthria *Difficulty in articulation of speech.*	Kugigimiza
dyschezia *Pain experienced during defecation.*	Imisonga mu kwikanira
dysentery *A severe form of diarrhea with blood and mucous in the stool.*	amacinya
dyshidrosis *Dysregulation of sweating*	Indwara yo kubira ivyuya
dysmenorrhea *Pain during menstruation.*	ububabare igihe ubutinyanka
dyspepsia *Indigestion.*	kwuzur inda
dysphagia *Difficulty in swallowing.*	Indwara yo kumira

67

English	Kirundi
dysphasia *Difficulty in speaking caused by cerebral dysfunction.*	Indwara yo kugigimiza
dyspnea *Difficult breathing.*	kuzibirwa impweno
dysuria *Difficulty or pain upon urination.*	Kubabwa kumukoyo
ear *The organ of hearing and balance.*	ugutwi
ear, the area behind and below the	imburukutwi
ear infection *General term referring to otitis media or otitis externa.*	Indwara yo mumatwi
ear, inner *Auris interna.*	Ugutwi kwimbere
ear, middle *Auris media.*	Ugutwi kwinyuma
ear-drum *Common term for tympanic membrane.*	ingoma y ugutwi
earache *Pain associated with the ear.*	ukuribwa mu matwi
earlobe *The soft, fleshy inferior portion of the pinna.*	igishato c'ugutwi
eat, to *To consume food.*	kurya
eating disorder *General term for pathologic eating habits.*	Kufungura nabi
ecchymosis *Skin discoloration caused by bleeding beneath the epidermis.*	Indwara yurukoba
echocardiogram *Use of ultrasound to evaluate the heart.*	gupima umutima
eclampsia *A maternal condition characterized by convulsions and hypertension that can lead to maternal and fetal death.*	Intandara zabagore bibungenze
ectopic pregnancy *A pregnancy that is not intrauterine.*	imbanyi iri inyuma y'igitereko
ectropion *Eversion of the eyelid, usually the lower lid.*	kuhenesha idzjicho
eczema *A medical condition exhibited by pruritic, red, scaly patches on the scalp, cheeks and extensor surfaces.*	izabana
edema *Extravascular fluid accumulation.*	ukububika amazi munsi y'urukoba
education *Instruction or guidance.*	amashure
efficacious *Effective.*	gikora neza
effort *Attempt or endeavor.*	akigoro
ejaculation *The emission of semen at the moment of sexual climax in a male.*	ugusuka intanga
elbow *The joint between the humerus and radius/ulna.(right elbow, left elbow)*	inkokora; nyamanyakawiri
elderly *Advanced in years.*	umusaza
elective *Non-urgent and not life-saving.*	kitihutirwa
elephantiasis *A condition caused by nematode parasites leading to lymphatic obstruction and limb or scrotal swelling.*	imisozi; umusozi
elephantiasis of the scrotum *A condition caused by nematode parasites leading to lymphatic obstruction scrotal swelling.*	imisuha
elixir *A medical solution.*	umuti
emaciated,to be *To be abnormally thin and weak.*	kunyunyuka
embryo *The term used to describe a fertilized ovum in the first 8 weeks of development.*	umwana akiri munda
emergence *Coming into prominence.*	ukuboneka
emergency *An urgent, life-threatening situation.*	ivyihutirwa cane
emergency room *A ward used for initial treatment of critical patients.*	mu ntabarimbabare
emesis,to have an *To vomit.*	kuruka
emollient *Having softening or soothing qualities.*	gitezura

English	Kirundi
emotion *An intense feeling.*	ibihagati
empathy *To be concerned for and share the feelings of another.*	ubucuti
emphysema *Abnormal enlargement of the airspaces distal to the terminal bronchioles.*	Indwara yamahaha
empty *Containing nothing.*	kigaragara
empyema *A collection of purulent material in a body cavity, usually referring to a thoracic empyema.*	igihute co mumahaha
encephalitis *Inflammation of the brain.*	mugiga yo mumutwe
encephalomyelitis *Inflammation of the brain and spinal cord.*	Mugiga yo mumutwe no mugiti cumugongo
encopresis *Involuntary defecation.*	kwiyitumako
end point *The last stage of a process.*	iherezo
end stage *Terminal stage. End stage cancer means there is no cure possible and death is imminent.*	intambwe yanyuma
endemic *When a disease is commonly found in a location or in a people group.*	ikiza
endometrium *The mucous membrane lining of the uterus.*	igihimba co mugitereko
endotracheal *Within the trachea.*	igihogohogo
endow, to *To supply or provide for.*	kuha
enema *A procedure involving insertion of fluid into the rectum.*	ukwitera umwino
enlargement *Becoming bigger.*	ukwagura
enormous *Very large.*	kinini cane
ensure, to *To make certain of.*	gusuzuma ko
ENT *Abbreviation for ears, nose and throat.*	Aamtwi, Amatwi nimihogo
enteral feeding *Nutrition supplied via the alimentary canal.*	kugaburirirwa mu mara
enterectomy *Surgical resection of part of the intestine.*	Kubaga amara
enteritis *Inflammation of the intestines.*	indwara yo mumara
enucleation *Surgical removal of a globe.*	kubaga utuvyimba two mumubiri
enuresis *Involuntary urination.*	indwara yo kwisobako usinziriye
enzyme *A compound that acts as a catalyst for reactions within cells as assists with digestion outside of cells.*	inkabuzo
eosinophil *A cell with eosin stain used to designate a type of leukocyte that is elevated during allergic reactions.*	Ubwoko bwabasoda bumubiri bita Eosinophil
epidemic *Ubiquitous development of an infectious disease.*	ikiza
epidemiology *The study of the incidence, development and control of disease.*	icigwa c'indwara z'ikiza
epidermis *The skin cells overlying the dermis.*	urukoba
epididymitis *Inflammation of the duct that moves sperm from the testis to the vas deferens. (unilateral testicular swelling)*	akakangavya
epidural *The space around the dura of the spinal cord.*	igihima curuti rwumugongo
epidural anesthesia *Injection of medication in the epidural space for pain control. Commonly used during childbirth.*	n'urushinge batera mu ruti rw'umugongo
epigastrium *The section of the abdomen that overlies the stomach.*	akameme
epiglottis *Tissue at the base of the tongue that covers the trachea when one swallows.*	akarimirimi

English	Kirundi
epilepsy *A condition associated with abnormal brain activity and exhibited by sudden, recurrent convulsions, sensory disturbances and loss of consciousness.*	intandara
epileptic seizure *A convulsion related to abnormal brain activity (as opposed to being precipitated by hypoglycemia.)*	umushikanuro; ikifube
epistaxis *Bleeding emanating from the nose.*	umwuna
equal *The same or uniform.*	hamwe
equilibrium *When opposing forces are in balance.*	bidasumbanye
equipment *Apparatus or instrument.*	ibikoresho
erosion *The gradual destruction of surface tissue.*	inkukura
error *Mistake or inaccuracy.*	ifuti
eructation *Belch or burp.*	amangati
eruption of pustules *Initial onset of a cluster of pustules.*	uruhere
erysipelas *An acute infection caused by Streptococcus pyogenes that causes fever along with swelling and inflammation. The infection frequently effects the face or one leg.*	Indwara yo kuvyimba ukuguru bita Erysipele mukinofunofu
erythrocyte *Called a red blood cell, it transports oxygen and carbon dioxide to and from the tissues.*	Abisirikare b umubiri
eschar *Dry, hard, dead tissue commonly seen with a chronic pressure ulcer or anthrax.*	ikiwuwitsi
esophagectomy *Surgical removal of the esophagus.*	Kubaga umuhogo
esophagitis *Inflammation of the esophagus.*	indwara yo mumuhogo
esophagus *The muscular tube that connects the throat to the stomach.*	igihogohogo; umuhogo
esophageal reflux *Regurgitation of the stomach contents into the esophagus.*	ikirungurira
essential *Crucial or necessary.*	gikuru
eunuch *A man who has been castrated.*	umuntu w'inkone
eustachian tube *The muscular canal that connects the tympanic membrane with the pharynx*	akaringoti ko mugutwi
evacuation *The emptying of an organ of fluids or gas.*	gusohora umwuka
evaluation *Assessment or evaluation.*	ukubara
eversion *To turn outward.*	gusohoka
every day *Each day.*	c'imisi yose
every *Each or all possible.*	hose
every other day *On alternate days.*	buri misi ibiri
evident *Obvious.*	kigaragara
eviscerate,to *The removal of bowels from the body.*	kumena inda
exacerbation *Worsening of an existing problem.*	kwunyuka
examination,medical *Assessment or evaluation.*	igipimo co kwa muganga
exanthema *A rash that accompanies a disease or fever.*	amahere
excess *Surplus or overabundance.*	igisaga
excrement *Feces.*	umusarani;amavyi
exfoliation *The shedding of scales.*	kubaga ibisebe vyo kurukoba
exhumation *To remove a dead body from a grave.*	kuzura
exomphalos *Umbilical hernia.*	iromba
exophthalmos *Protrusion of one or both eyeballs.*	Guturumbura amaso

English	Kirundi
exostosis *A bony prominence growing from the surface of a bone.*	akagufa kinyongera
exotropia *A type of strabismus that is characterized by the eyes turned outward.*	ubwoko bw Imirazi
expansion *Enlargement or increase in size.*	ukwagura
expect, to *To suppose or presume.*	gusamaza
expectorate,to *To expulsion of sputum associated with a cough.*	gucira
expiration date *The date when a medication should no longer be used.*	Itariki imiti iyopfirako
expire,to *To exhale.*	guhemuka
expire, to *To die.*	gucikana
exploratory laparotomy *Abdominal surgery with the intent of examining the abdominal contents.*	Kubaga munda
expulsion *Evacuation or elimination.*	ukwirukana
expulsion of placenta *Passage of the placenta out the cervix after childbirth.*	Isohoka ry Ingovyi
extend, to *To expand or stretch out.*	gukwegura
external *Outside of the body.*	uko umuntu aboneka
extremity *Refers to one arm or one leg.*	ukuboko canke ukuguru
extubation *The removal of a tube that was in a body orifice.*	Kusokora
exudate *The fluid, cells, and debris found in the tissues or a cavity (like pleural space) during inflammation.*	Imicafu y umubiri
eye discharge *Conjunctival discharge.*	Ibirashi
eye drops *Liquid applied to eyes for various medical problems.*	Amosozi
eyebrow *Supercilium.*	ikigohegohe
eyeglasses *Eye wear used for cosmetic or prescription purposes.*	ivyirori; amarori
eyelash *Each of the short hairs on the eyelid.(eyelashes)*	urugohe (ingohe)
eyelid *Palpebra.*	ikigohe
eye test *Catch all phrase for ophthalmologic examination.*	igipimo c'amaso
face *Anterior aspect of the head from the forehead to the chin.*	amaso;uruhanga
face presentation *Referring to the part of the body coming out of the cervix first during childbirth.*	Kuvuka atanguje amaso
failure, organ *The cessation of function of body organs.*	ukudakora kw'igihimba c'umubiri
faint *Weak and dizzy.*	ukuraba
faint,to *To lose consciousness.*	kuraba
fair *Equitable.*	bitarimwo
fallopian tubes *Either of a pair of long narrow ducts located in a female's abdominal cavity that transport the male sperm cells to the egg.*	uturingoti twimbuto
family	indimwe
family planning *Birth control.*	ugutandukanya imvyaro
fascia *The fibrous sheath enclosing a muscle or organ.*	inyama igize imitsi yo munda
fasting *Absence of caloric intake for a specified period.*	amapfungo
fat *A greasy or oiling substance naturally occurring in the body.*	amavuta
fatal *Lethal.*	gishikana ku rupfu
fatigue *Tiredness and exhaustion.*	uburuhe

71

English	Kirundi
favus *Tinea capitis caused by Trichopyton schoenleini.*	indwara y'uburima
fear, to have *Fright or trepidation.*	gutinya; kwikanga
febrile *Presence of an supraphysiologic temperature.*	umuriro; inyonko
febrile, to be *To have a fever.*	kururumba
fecal impaction *The presence of hard excrement in the rectum that requires manual removal.*	ukugumbiza
feces *Excrement.*	ususarani
feel better or get better *To have improved health symptomatically.*	imisuhuko
feel, to *To perceive or discern.*	kwumva
female *Feminine. (female nurse)*	-kazi (umuforomakazi)
feminine pad *Gauze specially designed to absorb menstrual flow.*	agaswime
femur *The long bone in the thigh.*	igufa ry'itako; umuwero
fertility *The ability of a person to contribute to contraception.*	ukurondoka kw'abantu
fester, to *To become infected.*	kuzana amashira
fetal distress *Term used to describe an abnormal heart rate or rhythm in a fetus indicating the need for urgent childbirth.*	umwana ahema nabi
fetal movements *Sensations by the mother of fetal activity.*	ugukina kwumwana
fetal position *Refers to how the fetus lies within the uterus.*	iyicara ry umwana
fetus *Medical term for the infant prior to birth.*	urusoro; imbuto
fever *A temperature above the normal range.*	inyonko; umururumbo
fibrin *An insoluble protein formed when fibrinogen is acted upon by thrombin.*	ubwoko bwinkabuyo
fibrosis *Connective tissue that is scarred and thickened after injury.*	inkovu ivyimvye
fibula *The smaller of two bones in the lower leg.*	umurundi
filiform *Threadlike.*	imeze nkinyuzi
finger *Any of the five digits on the hand.*	urutoke
finger, extra *Congenital 6th finger.*	indorerezi
fingernail *Thin horny plate over the dorsal aspect of the end of finger.*	urwara
fingertip *Distal aspect of a finger.*	ubusunwa bw'urutoke
firm *Hard or unyielding.*	kigumye
first aid *The initial treatment after an injury.*	ibikorwa vy'ubtabazi
fissure *A general term for a cleft or deep groove. An anal fissure, for example, is a small ulcer adjacent to the anus.(anal fissure)*	umugaga (utusaduke ku'ikiworo)
fist *When a person has their fingers clenched tightly to the palm.*	ikifunzi
fistula *An abnormal communication between two organs or an organ and the skin, as in rectovaginal fistula.*	ikirimba
flaccid *Limp. A term applied to an extremity one cannot move actively.*	uworoshi; kinyoganyoga
flail chest *The term used when one has multiple rib fractures causing a segment of the chest wall to move incongruently with the rest of the chest wall.*	kuvunika amagufa yo mu gikiriza
flare-up *A sudden worsening one's condition.*	kwaduka
flask *A narrow-necked container.*	agacupa

72

English	Kirundi
flat *Level or even; without bulges.*	igitega
flatfoot (to have) *Common term for pes planus.*	kugira ibirenge bibase
flatulence *The gas expulsed from the anus.*	imisuzi
flatus,to pass *To expel air from the anus.*	gusurira
flea *A small wingless insect that feeds on blood of mammals.*	imbaragasa
flex To bend.	gukonya
flow *Movement in a continuous stream.*	urugero
fluid intake *The amount of oral consumption plus the amount of intravenous fluids administered.*	ivyinjijwe mu mubiri amazi
fluke *Parasitic nematode worm; an example is Schistosoma.*	inzoka yo mu gitigu
flutter,atrial *Used to describe a cardiac rhythm disturbance, as in atrial flutter.*	indihagizi y'umutima
foam *A mass of small bubbles in a liquid.*	ifuro
fontanelle or fontanel *The space between the bones in the skull that are separate at birth.*	uruhorihori
food intake *Quantitative record of nutritional intake.*	ivyinjijwe mu mubiri
food *Nutrition.*	indya
food poisoning *Poisoning where the active agent is in the food.*	ukurwazwa n'indya zityoye
foot (sole of the foot) *The lower extremity distal to the ankle.*	ikirenge
foot and mouth disease *A contagious viral disease exhibited by oral and digital vesicles.*	isuna
foramen *An opening in a bone.*	Intoboro yigufa
foramen magnum *The hole in the skull that the spinal cord passes through.*	Intoboro yigufa ryo mumutwe
forceps *A surgical instrument, commonly called tweezers.*	Icuma co kubaga
forearm *Segment of the arm from the elbow to wrist.*	igice c'ububoko gifatanye n'urutugu
forehead *Section of the face from the hairline to the eyebrows.*	uruhanga
foreskin *Also called prepuce, the skin that naturally covers the glans but can be rolled back.*	urukoba rw'umutwe w'imvyarabibondo
former *Prior.*	mbere
forwards *Towards the front.*	imbere
fossa *A shallow depression.*	intoboro
fracture *A broken bone.*	imvune
fracture, comminuted *A broken bone where one segment overrides the other.*	Kuvunagurika kwamagufa
fracture, greenstick *A spiral fracture.*	Ivunika ryamagufa yabana
framboesia; yaws *An endemic tropical disease caused by Treponema pertenue.*	ibintoro
free from *Lacking or absent.*	aka
frenulum linguae *A fold of tissue extending from the floor of the mouth to the midline of the under part of the tongue.*	inkingi y'ururimi
frequency *Rate of occurrence.*	igarukagaruka
friable,to be *Easily reduced to powder.*	kuvungagurika
friction *Grating or rasping.*	umusyegenyo
frog *A tailless amphibian that is short with long hind legs for jumping.*	igikere
frontal *Referring to the anterior aspect, as in frontal lobe.*	kijanye n'uruhanga

73

English	Kirundi
frostbite *Local tissue destruction after exposure to cold.*	ubushe buvuye kubukanye
froth at the mouth, to *To have a mass of saliva with small bubbles in it coming out of the mouth.*	kugira ifuro ku munwa
froth *Covered with a mass of small bubbles.*	ifuro
frozen *Past participle of to freeze. Freeze: turn a liquid into a solid.*	gikonje
frozen shoulder *Common term for adhesive capsulitis.*	indwara yo murutugu
fungus *A spore-producing organism that feeds on organic matter.*	urwoba
furuncle *A painful erythematous nodule with a central core.*	ikirimba
gag,to *To choke or retch.*	kuniga
gait *The way one walks.*	amagizo
gallbladder *The organ adjacent to the liver that stores bile and secretes it into the duodenum.*	Indugu
gallop *An abnormal heart sound.*	isimbasimba
gallstone *Calculus produced in the bile duct or gallbladder.*	akabuye kaba mu mugende w'indurwe
gangrene *Tissue death from either impaired blood flow or an infection.*	inyama iwoze
gaping *Wide open.*	gitaburuye
gargle, to *To rinse one's mouth out and exhale through the liquid.*	kwinyugunyura
gastrectomy *Complete or partial surgical resection of the stomach.*	Kubaga umushishito
gastric *Referring to the stomach.*	kijanye n'umushishito
gastritis *Inflammation of the stomach.*	indwara y'umushihito
gastrocnemius *A large muscle in the lower leg, responsible for ankle plantar flexion, that is attached to the distal femur and achilles tendon.*	Umutsi womukuguru
gastroduodenal ulcer *A lesion in the mucosal lining of the stomach or duodenum.*	Indwara ya iriseri yo mumushishito
gastroenteritis *A bacterial or viral infection that leads to vomiting and diarrhea.*	indwara y'amara n'inda
gastrostomy *A surgical creation of an opening in the stomach.*	kubaga umushishito
gauze *A fabric used for dressing changes.*	uwuhomyi
gaze *Steady, intent look.*	uguhanga
gene *A unit of heredity that is passed on from parent to child.*	intunganyakaronda
general appearance *The overall look of a patient.*	Isura
general *Common or expected.*	kizwi hose
genital ambiguity *A disorder of sexual development in which the genitalia are not sufficiently developed to tell clearly if the person is male or female.*	bitumbiri
genital herpes *A sexually transmitted infection caused by herpes simplex.*	indwara zo mubihimba vyirondoka
genital wart *The common term for Condylomata acuminata.*	isununu mu ntantu
genitalia *Genitals.*	ibihimba vy'irondoka
genu valgum *A condition exhibited by the knees turning inward, commonly referred to as knock-knee.*	Imibango

English	Kirundi
genu varum *A condition exhibited by the knees turning outward, commonly referred to as bowleg.*	amaguru y'inkika
geriatrics *The study of the health of old people.*	ubuhanga bw'ukuvura abatama
germ *Microorganism.*	umugera w'indwara
German measles *(rubella) A contagious viral infection.*	ibihara
gestation *The development of a fetus from conception until birth.*	kuchukwa mimba
get up out of bed	Vyuka
giant *Huge or massive.*	kirekire cana rwose
giardiasis *A flagellate protozoa, Giardia lamblia, that causes diarrhea.*	Inzoka yo munda
giddiness *A tendency to fall or dizziness.*	kizunguzungu
gingival *Referring to the gums.*	Indwara yo mu bishinyi
gingivitis *Inflammation of the gums.*	indwara yo kuvyimba ibinyigishi; ividzjegezi
glance *A brief look at something.*	ururabwe
glans penis *The distal aspect of the penis.*	umutwe w'imboro; intini
glare *An angry stare.*	urutsure
Glasgow coma scale *A scale used to grade one's level of consciousness with a score of 3 being totally unresponsive and a score of 15 being normal.*	Igipimo c urugero rwubwenge bwindembe
glaucoma *A condition characterized by increased intraocular pressure.*	Indwara y amaso
glossectomy *Surgical resection of the whole or part of the tongue.*	kubaga ururimi
glossitis *Inflammation of the tongue.*	uwegendakanwa
glossodynia *Tongue pain.*	Umusonga wo kururimi
glottis *Essentially the vocal structure, including the true vocal cords and the opening between them.*	amarakaraka
glove *Covering for hand protection.*	ikirato c'intoke
glucagon *A pancreatic enzyme responsible for breakdown of glycogen to glucose.*	Inkabuzo yo mu rwagasha
glue *Plastic cements*	ubwome
gluteal or gluteus muscle *A paired set of three muscles, the gluteus maximus, medius and minimus, that all have origins in the ilium and insertions in the femur. (buttocks)*	ubwicariro
glycosuria *Presence of glucose in the urine.*	umukoyo urimwo isukari
gnosia *Ability to recognize things and people.*	Kumenya abantu nibintu
go to the doctor, to	genda kwa muganga
go to the hospital, to	genda ku bitaro
goiter *Swelling of the thyroid gland.*	umwingo
gold *Precious metal with atomic number of 79.*	inzahabu
gonad *A testis or an ovary.*	igihimba ntunganyambuto
gonorrhea *A sexually transmitted disease that is exhibited by purulent discharge from the vagina or penis.*	agaswende; mburugu
gonorrheal arthritis *A type of arthritis caused by the gram negative diplococcus Neisseria gonorrhoeae.*	Indwara yo mungingo
gonorrheal ophthalmia *An acute purulent conjunctivitis that can occur in neonates within 2-5 days of birth.*	indwara yo kubora mubihimba vy amaso

English	Kirundi
goose bumps *Cutis anserina.*	kumerereza
gout *Monosodium urate crystal deposition disease.*	ikisigo
gown *A sterile gown used during surgical procedures.*	ikanzu
graft *A piece of tissue surgically transplanted.*	kubaga urukoba
Graves' disease *A form of hyperthyroidism exhibited by a goiter and exophthalmos.*	indwara y umwingo
gravida *Pregnant woman.*	inda rikuze
greater than normal *Above normal.*	hejuru yibipimo fatiro
grief *Deep sorrow.*	intimba
groan *A deep inarticulate sound made due to pain or despair.*	induru
groin pull *A muscle strain in the inguinal region.*	gutabuka imitsi yo mw iteranirizo ry itako
groin *The genital region.*	ikiwuno
growth *The increase in physical size.*	ugukura
guarding *A symptom used to describe a patient resisting an examination because of severe pain; often seen in patients with peritonitis.*	umusonga wo munda
guinea worm *A parasitic nematode worm that, in cases of infection, lives under the skin, formally called Dracunculus medinensis.*	Inzoka yo kurukoba
gum *Gingiva.*	ikinygishi
gumboil *Swelling noted on the gingiva over a dental abscess.*	ikyekezi
gumma *A soft granulomatous tumor of the skin or cardiovascular system seen in tertiary syphilis.*	ikivyimba co kurukoba canke mu mutima bivuye ku ndwara ya mburugu
gunshot wound *An penetrating injury sustained from a bullet.*	igikomere cuwarashwe
gustatory agnosia *The loss of the sense of taste.*	indwara yo kutumva akanovera
gynecomastia *Enlargement of the breasts.*	indwara yo kuvyimba amabere
habit *A custom or inclination.*	ingeso
hair (of body) {axillary and pubic hair}	ubgoya {inzia}
hair (of head) {facial hair- beard}	umushatsi {ubwanwa}
half *Divided in two.*	igice
half-life *The time a drug decreases its effect in half over time.*	igice c umwanya
halitosis *Foul odor emanating from the mouth.*	ukunuka mu kanwa
hallucination *A perception that is not based on reality.*	indwara yo kwikanga
hamstrings *Tendons of the posterior thigh.*	imitsi ifata inyama zo kumaguru
hand *The upper extremity distal to the wrist.*	igikonjo
hand, dorsum *Back of hand.*	igikonjo
hand, left	ukubamfu
hand, palm of	ikiganza
hand, right	igikonjo ciburyo
hangnail *A loose piece of skin attached near the medial or lateral nail fold.*	inkecuru
Hansen's disease *Leprosy*	imibeme

English	Kirundi
hard of hearing,to be *Decreased sense of hearing.*	kwumva bihurugushwi
hard *Rigid or very firm.*	kigumye
harmless *Safe or benign.*	kitica
hazy *Cloudy.*	igipfungu
head	umutwe
head contusion, resulting in a superficial hematoma	inkavyi
head trauma *Any injury to the brain.*	uruguma rwo kumutwe
headache *Cephalgia.*	akahanzi
heal, to *To treat or to cure.*	gisigura gukiza indwara
healing *The process of becoming healthy again.*	ugukira
health center *A physical location where patients are treated.*	ivuriro rito
health *The state of being free of illness.*	amagara
healthy *In good health.*	c'amagara meza
hearing aid *A device that fits in the ear used to amplify sound.*	akuma gafasha kumva
hearing *Auditory perception.*	ukwumva
hearing test *Audiologic evaluation.*	igipimo c'amatwi
heart attack *Common term for myocardial infarction.*	gufatwa n'umutima
heart beat *A single contraction of the heart.*	indihaguzi
heart disease *Generic term generally meant to imply coronary disease.*	indwara y'umutima
heart murmur *An abnormal heart sound usually related to valvular disease.*	ikiriro
heart *Muscular organ that pumps blood thru the circulatory system.*	umutima
heart rate *Number or cardiac contractions per minute.*	urugero umutima utererako
heartburn *Synonym of pyrosis.*	ikirungurira
heat exhaustion *A condition that occurs secondary to prolonged exposure to high ambient temperature; it is exhibited by subnormal temperature, dizziness and nausea.*	kwuma mumubiri
heat stroke *A condition caused by excessive exposure to high ambient temperature; it is exhibited by dry skin, thirst, vertigo, muscle cramps and nausea. The three forms are heat exhaustion, heat cramps and sunstroke.*	umuyaya
heat *The quality of being hot.*	ubushuhe
heavy *Possessing great weight.*	kiremeye
heel *Proximal portion of the plantar aspect of the foot.*	igitsintsiri
heel-shin test (heel to knee to toe test) *A test of position sense and coordination; one moves the heel of one foot from the knee on the other foot down to the foot.*	igipimo co kuraba ko umurwayi wimitsi ashobora gutembereza agatsinstiri kuva kwivi gushika kukirenge iburyo n ibubamfu.
height *Distance between the bottom of the foot and top of the head.*	uburebure
hematemesis *Vomiting blood.*	kudahwa amaraso

English	Kirundi
hematochezia *Presence of blood in the excrement.*	amacyinya
hematoma *A mass containing blood.*	ikisumbano; ifufu
hematuria *The presence of blood in the urine.*	akasokoro
hemeralopia *Night blindness.*	amaso arirashye
hemiparesis *Unilateral muscle weakness (half the body).*	kutetemera igice cumubiri
hemiplegia *Paralysis of one side of the body.*	akasate
hemoglobin *An iron containing protein used for the transport of oxygen in blood.*	inkabuzo zigize amaraso
hemolysis *Breakdown of hemoglobin.*	kuyonga kwamaraso
hemopericardium *Abnormal presence of blood in the pericardium.*	gusanga amaraso mugasaho gapfuka umutima
hemophilia *A hereditary bleeding disorder characterized by hemarthroses and deep tissue bleeding as a result of absence of a coagulation factor such as factor VIII.*	Indwara yo kuva amaraso mumubiri
hemophthalmia *Bleeding within the eye.*	Indwara yo kuva amaraso mumaso
hemopoiesis *The production of blood cells from stem cells.*	Ihingurwa ry amaraso
hemoptysis *Expectoration of blood.*	Gukorora amaraso
hemorrhage,to have a *Bleeding from a damaged blood vessel.*	kuvra 'maraso
hemorrhoidectomy *Surgical excision of a hemorrhoid.*	Kubaga uturingoti two mugisusu
hemorrhoids *Engorgement of the veins in the anus or rectum.*	bawasiri
hemostasis *The control of bleeding.*	kuvura kwamaraso
hemothorax *The abnormal presence of blood in the pleural cavity.*	Kugira amaraso mugikiriza
hence *Thus.*	nico gituma
hepatectomy *Partial or complete surgical resection of the liver.*	kubaga igititgu
hepatitis *Inflammation of the liver. (hepatitis B)*	indwara y'igitigu (ingwara y'igitigu y'umugera wo mu murwi B)
hepatomegaly *Enlargement of the liver.*	kuvimba ikitigo
hereditary *That which is transmitted genetically*	c'akaronda
hermaphrodite *A person possessing gonadal characteristics of both sexes.*	magoremagabo
hernia *An abnormal bulge of bowel through muscle.*	ikihazi
hernia, epigastric *Hernia through the linea alba superior to the navel.*	ikirusu
hernia, inguinal *Protrusion of abdominal-cavity contents through the inguinal canal.*	irondo
hernia, umbilical *Protrusion of abdominal contents at the umbilicus.*	iromba
herniorrhaphy *The surgical repair of a hernia.*	Kubaga umusipa
herpes *A skin condition exhibited by formation of clustered vesicular lesions; herpes simplex is at times referred to, albeit incompletely, as herpes.*	umugera w urukoba
herpes zoster; shingles *A unilateral vesicular rash along one dermatome and caused by inflammation of a posterior nerve root by "the chicken pox virus".*	umugera wa virus y urukoba
heterogenous *That which originates outside the organism.*	Imvange, bivanze

English	Kirundi
hiccup *Involuntary spasm of the diaphragm with sudden closure of the glottis; this causes a characteristic cough.*	isevu
hidradenitis *Inflammation of a sweat gland. When there is purulent discharge it is called hidradenitis suppurativa.*	kubora kwuturingoti twamazi yo mumubiri
high altitude cerebral edema	ukuvyimba kwubwonko
high altitude pulmonary edema	ukuvyimba kwamahaha
high blood pressure *Elevated arterial blood pressure.*	umutima uratera vuba
high *Elevated.*	urugero rwo hejuru
hip *The lateral eminence of the pelvis from the waist to the thigh; it is formed by the iliac crest and greater trochanter.*	umusoso
hip replacement *Both joint surfaces are replaced by high density material such as plastic or metal.*	itako ry icuma
hirsutism *Abnormal growth on hair on a person's face and body.*	c'ubwoya
histamine *A chemical responsible for the reaction exhibited when a person has an allergic reaction.*	inkabuzo
histoplasmosis *A fungal pulmonary infection from bat and bird excrement.*	indwara y amahaha
HIV *Abbreviation for human immunodeficiency virus.*	umugera wa SIDA
hives *Urticaria*	indwara yurukoba iterwa nudukoko
hoarse *A rough, harsh sounding voice.*	ugusarara
hollow *An indentation.*	itako
homicide *When one person kills another.*	ukwica
hookworm *A parasitic infection of the family Strongylidae that can cause anemia.*	ankirositome
hordeolum *Inflammation of the sebaceous gland of the eye.*	indwara y uturingoti twamarira
hospital *Acute care medical/surgical facility.*	ibitaro
hospital discharge *To leave the hospital.*	gusohoka ibitaro
hot *Very warm.*	chaleur
human *Homo sapien.*	c'ubuntu
humerus *The long bone in the upper arm.*	ikizigira
hunchback *Synonym of kyphosis.*	inyonzo
hunger *A sense of discomfort caused by a lack of food.*	inzara
hydrate,to *To replenish fluid balance.*	kwongereza amazi
hydrocele *The accumulation of fluid in a body sac.*	indwara y udusaho twumubiri tuvyimbishwa n amazi
hydrocephalus *The excessive accumulation of cerebral spinal fluid in the brain causing enlargement of the head.*	igwirirana ry amazi mudusaho twubwonko
hydrophobia *Abnormal fear of water.*	gutinya amazi
hydrothorax *Accumulation of fluid within the thoracic cavity.*	igwirirana ry amazi mugikiriza
hygiene *Practices related to cleanliness.*	isuku
hymen *A membrane in the vagina.*	ince
hyperbaric *Use of gas at a higher than normal pressure.*	ikoreshwa ry impwemu kurugero runini
hyperglycemia *Higher than normal level of glucose in the blood.*	isukari nyinshi mu mubiri
hyperhidrosis *Excessive perspiration.*	kuwiza icyuya cane

79

English	Kirundi
hypermnesia *Unusually good memory.*	indwara yo kutibagira
hyperopia *Farsightedness.*	ukubona ibiri kure guza
hyperphagia *Excessive food ingestion.*	igisambo
hyperpigmentation, skin disease causing *General term to describe skin darkening.*	indwara y urukoba
hyperpnea *Abnormal increase in rate and depth of respiration.*	guhezagirika
hyperpyrexia *Fever.*	umuriro; ubushuhe
hypersalivation *Abnormal increase in salivation.*	irekwe
hypersensitivity *Abnormal increase in sensitivity.*	kugotwa
hypertension *Higher than normal blood pressure.*	umutima uratera vuba
hyperthermia *Fever.*	umuriro; ubushuhe
hypertrichosis *Excessive hair growth.*	ikura rirengeje urugero ry umushatsi
hyperventilation *Rapid and deep respirations.*	guhema cane
hypnotic *Sleep inducing agent.*	gusinziriza
hypogastrium *The area of the central abdomen located below the stomach.*	umusumbi
hypoglycemia *Abnormally low blood sugar.*	gukama isukari mumubiri
hypotension *Abnormally low blood pressure.*	umutima utera buhoro
hypothalamus *Located inferior to the thalamus it controls visceral activities, water balance, temperature and sleep.*	igihimba cubwonko
hypothermia *Lower than normal temperature.*	gukanya
hypoxia *Diminished oxygen content.*	kubura impemu
hysterectomy *Surgical removal of the uterus.*	kubaga igitereko
hysteria *A psychological condition exhibited by uncontrolled emotion or exaggerated manifestations.*	uwusazi
iatrogenic *A problem caused by medical treatment.*	inkurikizi y imiti
ichthyosis *A congenital anomaly exhibited by excessively dry, thick skin.*	indwara yo ku kwuma kurukoba
icterus *Yellowing of the skin and sclerae because of excess bilirubin.*	amaso atukura
identical twins *Twins from the same zygote.*	amahasa biteye kumwe
idiopathic *Relating to a disease with an unknown cause.*	indwara itazwi ikiyitera
ileum *The third portion of the small intestine, extending from the jejunum to the ileocecal valve.*	impindura
iliopsoas *A group of muscles inserting on the anterior aspect of the lesser trochanter of the femur.*	isohoro
ilium *The large bone at the superior aspect of the pelvis which is present bilaterally.*	igufa ry'ikiwuno
illiterate *Unable to read or write.*	atazi gusoma n'ukwandika
illness *Diseases, sickness or malady.*	indwara
immune *Being resistant to an infection.*	kijanye n'inkingiramubiri
immunization *A medication given to provide immunity.*	urucandago
immunodeficiency *An inadequate immune response.*	ugukora nabi kw' inkingiramubiri
impaction, tooth *A tooth that does not erupt because adjacent teeth prevent it.*	Ibihatane
impairment *A specific disability.*	ubumuga

English	Kirundi
imperforate *Lack of an opening. An infant with an imperforate anus has a congenital defect with no anal opening.*	gusiba y'intoboro
impervious *Not affected by.*	kitanyengetera
impetigo	indwara yurukoba
implementation *The process of putting a plan into effect.*	gushira mu ngiro
impotence *Inability to act or inability to achieve a penile erection.*	ukutakira inkomezi mpuzabitsina
inarticulate *Indistinct speech.*	imvugo itarongorotse
incision *An intentional surgical cut in the skin.*	ururasago
incisor *Sharp-edged tooth; humans have four incisors.*	amarwi
incoherent *Absence of intelligible speech.*	kitumvikana
incontinence *Inability to control urination.*	ukwisobako
incoordination *Absence of smooth, efficient body movement.*	kubira y'uwuringanizi
increment *An increase on a fixed scale.*	ivyongewe
incubator *A warming device for infants.*	icuma kibundikira abana
indeed *As a matter of fact.*	ata nkeka
indigenous *Naturally occurring.*	umusangwabutaka
indolent *1. Causing little pain. 2. Slow healing ulcer.*	afise ubunebwe
induce, to *Facilitated. When referring to labor, it means medication was given to assist in delivery of the fetus. (induce labor)*	kujijura (gutuma imbanyi ivuka ningoga)
induced abortion *Surgical or medical evacuation of the fetus.*	gukoroza imbanyi
induration *An area that is abnormally hard.*	umubiri uvyimvye
indwelling catheter *Continuous use tube usually referring to a tube in the urinary bladder.*	umuringoti binjiza mumubiri wo kwa muganga
inebriation *Intoxication with drugs or alcohol.*	ukuborewa
ineffective *Unsuccessful or inefficient.*	uburyo ataco bushikanako
inertia *The tendency to remain unchanged.*	uwuremere
inevitable, to be *Not preventable.*	kutatanya
infancy *Early childhood.*	ubuyoya
infant *Newborn.*	uruyoya; uruhinja
infarct *Referring to dead tissue.*	umubiri uboze
infection *A contagious disease.*	uwuhuguto.
infectious disease *Any disease or condition considered contagious.*	kwandukiza
inferior *The lower aspect.*	hasi
inflammation *Localized redness, excessive warmth and swelling.*	ubuvyimbe
influenza *Viral infection causing fever, muscle aches and catarrh. (hemophilus influenza B)*	muhure (ibicurane vyo mu muri wa B)
infuse,to *The injection of fluid into tissue or a vein.*	gutera urushinge
ingestion *The intake of food or liquid orally.*	kurya canke kunywa
ingrown nail *Also referred to as onychocryptosis.*	indwara y inzaara
inguinal *Referring to the groin.*	y'imisumbi
inhalation *The act of breathing in.*	uwuhemyi
inject,to *The act of a needle being inserted into a body. (given injection)*	gutera urushinge

81

English	Kirundi
injure, to be *To hurt or to wound.*	gukomereka
injury, to have an *To have a wound.*	kukomera
injury *A wound, abrasion or contusion.*	ikikomere; ikisebe
inoculation *Injection with a vaccine to provide immunity.*	icandaga
insane *A term not used in formal medical evaluations that when used by a layperson means a serious mental illness.*	arwaye mu mutwe
insanity *Referring to a serious mental illness.*	ubusazi
insect bite	umusemoro
insertion *The act of inserting something.*	ukugobeka
inside *Inner part, center.*	imbere mu
insidious *A slow, gradual and harmful advancement.*	kibangamye cane
insomnia *Sleeplessness.*	kutapata usingizi; ukubura itiro
inspiration *Drawing in a breath.*	ukwinjiza impwemu
instep *The medial aspect of the foot between the ankle and the ball of the foot.*	hedzjuru ry'ikirenge
insulin *A hormone produced by the pancreas and synthetically to control blood glucose levels.*	Inkabuzo yo mu rwagasha
intensive care *Vigorous treatment of the acutely ill.*	kuvurwa cane
intercostal *Area between the ribs*	hagati y amagufa yomugikiriza
intermittent *Occurring at irregular intervals.*	urugenda rw'imirindi
internal *Situated on the inside.*	y'imbere
interval *An intervening time.*	umwanya
intestinal obstruction *Blockage of the intestine by mass or volvulus.*	kuzib'inda
intestines *A general term used for the section of bowel from the stomach to the anus.*	amara
intestine, large *Portion of the bowel from the ileocecal valve to the rectum.*	uwura w'amata
intestine, small *The portion of the small bowel extending from the pylorus to the ileocecal valve.*	uwura w'amayoge
intraabdominal abscess *A collection of pus in the abdomen.*	igihute co munda
intraabdominal *Within the abdominal cavity.*	c'imbere y'inda
intracerebral *Within the cerebrum.*	mubwonko
intracranial *Within the cranial vault.*	c'imbere w'umutwe
intramuscular *Within a muscle.*	co mu nyama
intraosseous *Within a bone.*	mumagufa
intrauterine contraceptive device (IUD) *A device used to physically prevent the implantation of a fertilized ovum.*	akuma ko kuringaniza uruvyaro ko mu gitereko
intrauterine *Within the uterus.*	c'imbere mu gitereko
intravenous *Within a vein.*	gica mu mutsi w'amaraso
inversion *Turning inward.*	uwuhinduzi
involuntary movement *Movement not controlled consciously.*	ugukakaza vitari 'vigirankana
ipsilateral *On the same side.*	hahandi nyene
iris *The anterior portion of the vascular tunic of the eye.*	imbonero
iron *An element found in hemoglobin.*	icuma
iron-deficiency anemia *A microcytic anemia.*	gukama amaraso
irrelevant *Not pertinent.*	kitagira ico gifasha

English	Kirundi
irritable bowel syndrome *A gastrointestinal syndrome characterized by bloating, gas, constipation and diarrhea without an identified cause.*	ikisigo
ischemia *Inadequate blood supply to a part of the body.*	ugupfa kwinyama yumubiri kubera iura ry amaraso
ischium *The inferoposterior portion of the pelvis.*	rimwe mumagufa agize ikiyunguyungu
isolation ward *A ward where patients with infectious disease are housed.*	icumba vyahariwe abarwaye indwara zandukira
itch *A sensation that makes one want to scratch.*	ubusasate
itch, to *To have a sensation of pruritis.*	guhurira
jaundice of the newborn *A form of jaundice seen in newborns in the first two weeks of life; also called icterus neonatorum.*	ukubenja kwamaso y abana
jaundice *Yellowing of the sclerae and skin because of excessive bilirubin in the blood.*	uwutukure
jaw *Mandible.*	amashanya
jejunum *The portion of the small intestine from the end of the duodenum to the ileum.*	uwara w'amata
jock itch *Pruritus caused by tinea cruris.*	Indwara y urukoba
joint *Articulation of two adjacent bones.*	ingingo; urugingo
jugular vein (s) *Includes the internal, external and anterior jugular veins.*	umutsi utwara amaraso wo kwizosi
jugular venous distension *Enlarged jugular veins caused by high pulmonary capillary pressure.*	kuvyimba kwumutsi utwara amaraso wo kwizosi
juxta-articular *Positioned near a joint.*	hafi y iteranirizo ry amagufa
kala-azar *A disease caused by Leishmania donovani that is exhibited by weight loss, fever, anemia and hepatosplenomegaly.*	indwara bita leishmaniose
Kaposi sarcoma *Typically seen in AIDS patients, it is characterized by cutaneous reddish-purple macules and plaques.Also called multiple idiopathic hemorrhagic sarcoma.*	kanseri y urukoba
keloid *Hypertrophic scar tissue that forms after a minor cut or surgical procedure.*	indwara y inkovu
keratin *A protein found in the skin, hair, nails and enamel of the teeth.*	ubwoko kw inkabuzo
kick, to *To strike an object with one's foot.*	gutera umugere
kidney *One of two glandular organs that form urine.*	ifigo
knee *The joint at the distal femur and proximal tibia.*	ivi
knee elbow position *Knees and elbows are on the table and the chest is in the air.*	gupfukamisha amavi n inkokora
kneecap *Common term for patella.*	pia ya mguu; iyitfu m'ivi
kneel,to *Being on one's knees as in the prayer position.*	gupfukama
knock knees *Common term for genu valgum.*	ubwoko bw imibango
knot *A fastening made by tying a suture, for instance.*	ipfundo
known,to be *Recognized or familiar.*	kumenyekana
knuckles *Metacarpophalangeal joints or finger joints when the fist is closed.*	ingingo y'urutoke
kwashiorkor *A form of malnutrition from inadequate protein intake.*	indwara yo gufungura nabi
kyphosis *Abnormal outward curvature of the spine.*	inyonzo

83

English	Kirundi
lab result *The data obtained from a laboratory test.*	inyishu zibipimo
labia majora *The folds of skin forming the lateral borders of the pudendal cleft.*	umukoba
labia minora *The folds of skin enclosed in the pudendal cleft within the labia majora.*	umusino
labium *Referring to any lip shaped structure.*	umunwa
labor onset *The time when a pregnant woman begins uterine contractions in the process of childbirth.*	kuryarisha
labor pains *The intermittent pain associated with uterine contractions.*	ibise
labor, pre-term *Onset of labor prior to the expected date of birth.*	kuhurutura; kukorar'inda
laboratory test	gupima inyubakwa itunganirizwamwo ibipimo
laceration *An injury that is a cut/slice in the skin.*	ikihoro
lacrimal fluid *Fluid secreted by the lacrimal gland.*	amasozi
lacrimal *Referring to the secretion of tears.*	igihimba gihingura amosozi
lacrimation *The secretion of tears.*	kuva 'masozi
lactation *The secretion of milk from mammary glands.*	uguhembera
lagophthalmos *Characterized by the inability to close the eyelid completely over the eye.*	indwara yo kutasinzira (kutungara amaso)
lancet *A small sharp instrument used to obtain a drop of blood for testing.*	agashinge
laparotomy *A surgical incision of the abdomen.*	Kubaga munda
laryngectomy *Surgical removal of the larynx.*	kubaga mumuhogo
laryngitis *Inflammation of the larynx.*	ivyimba ry'umuhogo
laryngospasm *Sudden, involuntary muscle contraction of the larynx.*	indwara yo mumagage
laryngotomy *Surgical creation of an opening in the larynx.*	kubaga kumuhogo
larynx *A hollow muscular structure that contains the vocal cords.*	ikihogohogo
last *Final.*	c'impera
late *A time later than expected.*	cacerewe
lateral *Referring to the side of the body.*	co mu mbavu
laugh, to	gutwenga
laxity *A description of a joint that is loose.*	ugufata
layer *A stratum or thickness.*	uwuriri
lead *An element with an atomic number of 82.*	icunyunyu ca Plomb
lead poisoning *The ingestion of lead, exhibited in severe cases by paralysis, encephalopathy, purple gingiva, and colic.*	kurwazwa n ubumara bwicunyunyu cam Plomb
leakage *Unintentional escape of gas or fluid.*	gusohoka
learning *The intentional acquisition of knowledge.*	ubumenyo buhanitse
leech *An annelid used in some tropical regions for drawing out blood; they have an anticoagulant effect locally and have been attached to digits of persons with acute peripheral ischemia.*	umureberebe
left	ibumoso;ibubamfu
left-handed *The preference of using the left hand for common tasks.*	abangutse ibamfu

84

English	Kirundi
leg *One of two lower extremities.*	ukuguru
leishmaniasis *A condition caused by a flagellate protozoan parasite that is exhibited by visceral or dermatologic manifestations.*	indwara y urukoba bita leishmaniose
length *The end to end measurement.*	uburebure
lengthen,to *To make or become longer.*	gutahura
lens *The transparent chamber between the posterior chamber and the vitreous body.*	imbonero
leprosy *A contagious disease caused by Mycobacterium leprae that causes insensate papules and disfiguration.*	imibembe
less *A smaller amount.*	bike kurusha
lethal *Deadly.*	cica
lethal dose *The amount of a drug required to cause death.*	igipimu cumuti ushobora kwica
lethargy *Absence of energy.*	itaro irasa n'urufu
leukocyte *A white blood cell.*	ibice nkingiramubiri biri mu bigeze amaraso
leukorrhea *Thick white vaginal discharge.*	uruziri
lice *Plural for louse, a small parasite that lives on the skin. Pediculus humanus capitis is a head louse.*	amada
life expectancy *The length of time a person is anticipated to live.*	imyaka yo kubaho
life-threatening *Potentially fatal.*	kibangamye
lifetime *Duration of a person's life.*	ubuzima bwose
lift, to *Raise to a higher level.*	gukiriza
ligament *A band of fibrous connective tissue that connects two bones or cartilage.*	inyama y'imidzimidzi
ligature *A thread used to tie a vessel.*	imisurusura
light *Illumination, bright.*	umuco
light *Not heavy.*	gihwahutse
likelihood *The probability or feasibility.*	ugushoboka
lip *The fleshy tissue surrounding the mouth.*	umunwa
lip, lower *Labium inferius oris.*	umunwa wo hasi
lip, upper *Labium superius oris.*	umunwa wo hejuru
lipoma *A benign tumor consisting of fat cells.*	ikivyimba
lisping *A speech problem in which "s" and "z" are pronounced "th".*	ubureve
liver *A large glandular organ in the right upper quadrant that functions in digestive processes, as well as, neutralizing toxins.*	igitigu
liver abscess *A localized collection of pus in the liver.*	Igihute co mugitigu
localize,to *Toward one point or area.*	kudomako urutoke
loculated *Divided into small cavities.*	igabanywa mudusaho twinshi
long-acting *Referring to a drug with long lasting effects.*	umuti ukora umwanya muremure
long-standing *Having existed for a long time.*	Kuramba
longevity *Long life.*	uburambe
longsighted *Synonym of hyperopia.*	afise amaso y'ubusaza
loose *Not tight.*	kiregarega

English	Kirundi
loss of consciousness *Unresponsive to verbal and tactile stimuli.*	kutamenya
lots of *An abundance of.*	vyinshi
low back pain *Pain in the lumbar region.*	uwuwawazi w'ikiwuno; ikinyamukinya
lower extremity edema *Interstitial edema of the legs.*	adindye amaguru
lubricant *Emollient.*	corosha
lumbago *Pain in the region of the lumbar spine.*	uwuwawazi w'ikiwuno; ikinyamukinya
lumbar *Referring to the spinal region inferior to the thoracic spine.*	amafinya
lump *A protuberance.*	incavyi
lung *One of a pair of respiratory organs.*	ihaha
lymph *A transparent and sometimes opalescent fluid that flows in the lymph channels.*	amazi asa n amata yo mumubiri,ahingura abasirikare bumubiri
lymph node *An area of organized lymphatic tissue.*	intege
lymphangitis *Inflammation of the lymph vessels.*	isumbi
lymphocyte *A white blood cell produced by the lymph tissue.*	abasirikare b umubiri
lymphoma *A malignant disease of the lymph system, Hodgkin's lymphoma for example.*	ikivyimba
macrocheilia *Abnormally large lips.*	iminwa minini
macrodactyly *Abnormally large digits.*	intoke ndende
macroencephaly *Having an abnormally large head.*	indwara y umutwe munini
macroglossia *Abnormally large tongue.*	indwara y ururimi runini
macula solaris *Formal medical term describing a freckle.*	indwara zo kumubiri
mad cow disease *Bovine spongiform encephalopathy, a disease that cause cerebral degeneration exhibited by ataxia.*	indwara yo mu bwonko
madness *Common term for insanity.*	uwusazi
magnet *A piece of iron with atoms ordered to make it magnetic.*	umukunzi
malaise *A vague feeling of discomfort or unease.*	unyongonyo
malaria *A condition caused by a protozoan of the genus Plasmodium. It is transmitted by mosquitos and is exhibited by fever, chills, headache. In the severe form it can lead to convulsions, increased ICP and death.*	inyonko
malignancy *Tendency of a tumor to invade normal tissue.*	ikivyimba
malinger,to *To feign illness.*	kwirwaza
malleolus *A bony protrusion on medial and lateral aspect of each ankle.*	ikirenge cy'ukuguru
malnutrition *Lack of appropriate nutrition.*	ukubura ingaburo
mammary *Referring to the breast.*	kijanye n'amabere
mammogram *X ray imaging of the breasts to look for breast cancer.*	gusuzumisha amabere imishwarara (x)
man *Male human.*	umugabo
management *The process of dealing with things or people.*	ugutunganya
mandatory *Obligatory.*	c'itegeko
mandible *The lower jaw.*	amashanya
mania *A mental disorder exhibited by hyperexcitability, delusions and euphoria.*	uwusazi; uwuzeze

English	Kirundi
marasmus *Progressive weight loss and emaciation.*	indwara yo kufungua nabi
marijuana *Cannabis.*	urumogi
marital counseling *Therapy aimed at marriage reconciliation.*	guhuza imiryango
marital status *Single versus married status.*	urwego rwumuntu. Ingaragu vs uwubatse
marriage *The formal union of a man and a woman.*	ubukwe
marsupialization *Creation of a surgical pouch.*	ubuhinga bwo kubaga
mass *Tumor.*	ikivyimba
mastectomy *Surgical resection of one or both breasts.*	kubaga ibere
masticate,to *To chew.*	guhekenya
mastitis *Inflammation of the breast.*	indwara y amabere
mastodynia *Breast pain.*	umusonga mw ibere
mastoid *Referring to the mastoid process.*	igufa ro mumusaya, rir inyuma y ugutwi
matching *Corresponding in pattern or style.*	uguhuza
maternity *Area of the hospital where women deliver babies.*	mw'ivyariro
mattress *A fabric case filled with material, used for sleeping.*	imatera
maxilla *The upper jaw that also forms the inferior portion of the orbit and part of the nose.*	agasendabageni
meaningless *Having no significance.*	kitumvikana
measles *A childhood viral, infectious disease exhibited by rash and fever.*	agasama
meatus, urethral *Orifice at the entrance of the urethra.*	umwenge
meconium *The first newborn feces which are green.*	umwanda mukuru wa mberew umwana
medial *Situated toward the midline.*	co hagati
mediastinum *The thoracic area between the lungs.*	mu gikiriza
medication *A substance used for medical treatment.*	umuti ; uwuruzi
medicine *A substance used for medical treatment or the art and science of healing patients.*	umuti
medicine, to get	kuronka imiti
megacolon *Abnormal enlargement and dilatation of the colon.*	indwara y amara
meibomian cyst *An enclosed fluid collection along a sebaceous gland of the eyelid.*	utuherehere
melancholia *Profound sadness.*	intuntu
melanoma *Malignant cancer, typically found in the skin.*	kanseri
melena *The passage of black, tarry stools indicative of upper gastrointestinal bleeding.*	kwituma amaraso
melitis *Inflammation of the cheek.*	indwara y amatama
member *Referring to an extremity (arm or leg).*	ukuwuku/ukuguru
memory *Ability to remember.*	uwukumbutsi
menarche *The time of the initial menstrual period.*	ubutinyanka y'icambere
meningeal *Referring to the dura mater, arachnoid and the pia mater.*	mu bwonko
meningitis *Inflammation of the meninges exhibited by fever, photophobia, nuchal rigidity and in severe cases coma and convulsions.*	mugiga
meniscus *A thin cartilage between joint surfaces.*	inyama yo mungingo y amagufa

English	Kirundi
menopause *The time when menstruation ceases.*	uguca imvyaro
menorrhagia *Abnormally large amount of menstrual blood.*	ubutinyanka cane
menses *The blood and other material expelled from the uterus during menstruation.*	ubutinyanka
menstrual cramps	ubutinyanka bubabaza
menstruation *Synonym of menses.*	ubutinyanka
menstruation, to have	kuja mu kwezi
mental *Cognitive or psychological.*	co mu bwenge
mention, to *Refer to or allude to.*	kuhamagara
metacarpophalangeal *Referring to the metacarpus and the phalanges.*	kijanye n'amagufa y'ikiganza
metatarsal *Referring to any of the metatarsal bones.*	kijanye n'amagufa y'amano
metrorrhagia *Uterine bleeding in normal amounts but at irregular intervals.*	kuva amaraso mu gitereko
microcephalic *A congenital deformity exhibited by an abnormally small head.*	indwara y ubwonko buto
micrognathia *Abnormally small maxilla or mandible.*	ubumuga bwamagufa yo mumisaya
microscope *A instrument used to magnify and view small objects.*	rugagamisha
micturate,to *Synonym of to urinate.*	kunyara
midwife *A person trained to assist in childbirth.*	umuvyazi
migraine *An episodic, unilateral headache accompanied by nausea.*	umutwe w'uruhande rumwe
mild *Slight, nominal.*	coroshe
milestone *An event indicative of a certain stage of development.*	intambwe ishimishije
minute *Something very small.*	kanzuya
mirror *A device used for reflecting an image.*	icirori
miscarriage *Spontaneous abortion.*	ukuruhira ubusa
mite fever *Synonym of typhus fever.*	tifoyide
moist *Damp or humid.*	kibomvye
molar tooth *Any of the most posterior teeth bilaterally which includes 8 deciduous and usually 12 permanent teeth.*	ijigo
monitor *A person that observes a process or a monitoring device.*	ikiyo
monocyte *A leukocyte with an oval nucleus and grey cytoplasm.*	Ubwoko bwabasoda bumubiri
monodiplopia *Double vision in only one eye.*	indwara yo kubona ibintu bibiri mwijisho rinwe
mononucleosis *An infectious disease exhibited by malaise and lymphadenopathy.*	indwara yo gusomana
monoplegia *Paralysis of a single limb.*	ku tetemera uruhande rumwe
mons pubis *The prominence over the symphysis pubis in a female caused by a fat pad.*	umusimbi
morbidity *The state of disease.*	umubabaro
morgue *A room where deceased patients are housed until sent to a funeral home.*	uburuhukiro
moribund *Near death.*	ari mu gupfa
morning sickness *Nausea associated with pregnancy.*	ukuzinduka uradahwa

English	Kirundi
mosquito net *A fine mesh fabric hung over a bed as a mosquito repellent.*	umusegetera
motion sickness *Nausea associated with travel.*	ukunyinganga uradahwa
motor *Referring to muscles.*	imisoso igize umubiri
mourning *A period of grieving.*	ikiriyo
mouth *The orifice on the lower part of the face.*	akanwa
mouthful *To take a large quantity of something in one's mouth.*	gutamira
mucous *A substance secreted by mucous membranes.*	umurenda
mucous plug *A mass of mucous and cells that forms in the cervical canal during pregnancy.*	ururenduka
multigravida *A woman who has been pregnant more than once.*	umuvyeyi amaze kwibungenga kenshi
multipara *A woman with more than one live births.*	umuvyeyi afise imvyaro nyinshi
mumble, to *To speak quietly and indistinctly.*	kwidedomba
mumps *A contagious viral disease that is exhibited by parotid swelling and puts males at risk for sterility. Also called epidemic parotitis.*	amasambambwika
muscle *A band if fibrous tissue that can contract.*	inyama
muscle weakness *Decreased muscular function.*	intege nke y'imidzi
muscle, abdominal	imitsi yo munda
muscle, biceps	imitsi yo kukuboko
muscle, calf	ifundo
muscle, deltoid	umutsi wo kurutugu
muscle, intercostal	imitsi yo mugatuntu
muscle, latissimus dorsi	ubwoko bw umutsi
muscle, oblique	ubwoko bw umutsi
muscle, pectoral	ubwoko bw umutsi wo mugikiriza
muscle, quadriceps	ubwoko bw umutsi wo kwitako
muscle, trapezius	ubwoko bw umutsi wo mumugongo
mute *Refraining from or being speechless.*	ikirangi
myalgia *Muscle pain.*	imisonga yo mu misoso
mycosis *A disease caused by a fungal infection.*	isi
myelitis *Inflammation of the spinal cord.*	indwara y umugongo

English	Kirundi
myocardial infarction *The death of myocardial tissue as a result of an interruption in flow to the region supplied by a coronary vessel.*	gufatwa n'umutima
myocardium *The middle layer of the heart wall.*	igihimba cumutima
myopia *Nearsightedness.*	kutawona kure
myositis *Inflammation of muscle tissue.*	indwara y imitsi
nail *The hard surface on the dorsal surface of the toes or fingers.*	urwara
nail matrix or nail bed *The area of the corium on which the nail rests.*	imirero y'uwara
name *A word by which a person is known.*	izina
nap *A brief sleep or catnap.*	umusanzi w'inzu
nappy *Diaper*	ikiremo cy'umwana; intutu
narcissism *Abnormally excessive self-interest.*	kwikunda cane
nasal bone	umusikati
nasal mucus *Secretions coming from the nose.*	ikisero
nasogastric tube *A tube that is inserted into the nose with the distal tip in the stomach; it is used for irrigation or drainage of gastric contents.*	umurinoti wo gushira mumushishito
nasopharyngeal *Referring to the nose and pharynx.*	mumazuru n imihogo
nasopharynx *The part of the pharynx which lies superior to the soft palate.*	mumazuru n imihogo
nausea *A feeling that one wants to vomit.*	ikirungurira; iseseme
navel *Umbilicus.*	umukondo
near *In close proximity.*	hafi
nebulizer *A device used for transforming a liquid into a fine mist for inhalation as in nebulized albuterol for an acute exacerbation of asthma.*	icuma gihingura umuti wo mumahaha
neck *The part of the body that connects the body to the head.*	izosi
neck, back of (nape) *Posterior aspect of the neck.*	igikanu
necropsy *Synonym of autopsy.*	ugusuzuma umuvyimba
necrosis *The death of most of the cells of the affected part.*	kubora kwigihimba cumubiri
need *A want or obligation.*	ubukene
needle biopsy *Use of a needle to aspirate body contents for microscopic or pathologic examination.*	urushinge rwo gupimisha
needle holder *A surgical instrument used to grasp a needle during suturing.*	Umukasi wo gushona
needle *The slender cylindrical device attached to a syringe.*	urushinge
negative *Contrary or opposing.*	kutagend\a neza kitarico
nematode *An endoparasite belonging to the class of the Nemathelminthes including roundworms and threadworms.*	inzoka zo munda
neonate *The term for a newborn infant for the first four weeks.*	uruyoya; umwana mutoyi
nephrectomy *Surgical removal of a kidney.*	kubaga ifyigo

English	Kirundi
nephritis *A general term meaning inflammation of a kidney that is further categorized depending on the associated pathology.*	indwara y amafzigo
nephrolithiasis *A calculus in the kidney.*	iwuye ry'isare
nephrolithotomy *Surgical removal of a renal calculus.*	Kubaga utubuye two mu mafyifo
nephrotomy *Surgical incision of the kidney.*	kubaga amafyigo
nerve *A fibrous band made up of axons and dendrites that connects the nervous systems with other organs.*	umudzi
neurapraxia *Paralysis from nerve injury but no degeneration of the nerve.*	kudadarara umubiri
neurectomy *Excision of a section of a nerve.*	kubaga umutsi nsoza bwenge
neuritis *Inflammation of a nerve.*	indwara y imitsi nsoza bwenge
neurology test	gupima ubwonko n'imitsi (gupima icumvirizo)
neuropathy *Structural of pathologic changes of the peripheral nervous system.*	indwara y imitsi nsoza bwenge
neurosurgery *Surgery of the brain or spinal cord.*	kubaga ubwonko canke uruti rw umugongo
neutrophil *A polymorphonuclear leukocyte.*	ubwoko bw abasirikare b umubiri
nevus *A benign, well-circumscribed growth of tissue of congenital origin.*	isununu
next *The following or upcoming.*	gikurikira
night blindness *Common term for nyctalopia, it refers to low vision with reduced illumination, often seen with Vitamin A deficiency.*	amaso arirashye
night sweats *Profuse sweating at night occurring with tuberculosis among other conditions.*	kubira icuya n'ijoro
nightmare *An unpleasant or frightening dream.*	umwikanzi
nipples *The small projections on the breast thru which milk is secreted in females.*	amasonzi
nocturia *Urination at night.*	gusoba n'ijoro
nocturnal *Referring to events that happen at night.*	w'ijoro
nodule *A small node in the skin of up to 1cm and in the lung up to 3cm.*	ikifundo
non-rebreather mask *A type of oxygen mask used to deliver a higher oxygen concentration.*	igihemesho co kwa muganga
nonpitting edema *Subcutaneous swelling that cannot be indented with compression.*	kuvyimba amaguru
noon *The 12 o'clock mid-day hour.*	amashoka
nose *The midface protuberance used for smelling and breathing.*	izuru
nose, blow the	gupfuna
nosebleed *Common term for epistaxis.*	umwuna; ikicyurane
nose, bridge of	umwiriri
nose, tip of the *Distal aspect of the nose.*	umwiriri
nostril *One of two openings in the nose used for air passage.*	umwenge y'izuru; itondi
nulligravida *A woman who has never been pregnant.*	umugore ataratwara inda
nullipara *A woman who has never given birth.*	umugore ataravyara
numbness *Decreased sensation to tactile stimuli.*	ikizimgami; uworohe

91

English	Kirundi
nurse *A person trained to care for the sick.(female nurse)*	umuforomo (umuforomokazi)
nurse, to *To suckle or feed a baby at the breast.*	kwonka; kwonsa
nursing care, to give *The assessment and treatment provided by nurses.*	kuvungavunga
nutrition *The process of supplying food needed for growth.*	y'ukurisha
obesity *Having a body mass index over 30kilograms/meters squared.*	ikida
obsolete *No longer in use; antiquated.*	catayigihe
obstructed *To be blocked or halted.*	hugaye
obtuse *Rather insensitive or hard to understand.*	ikizeze; wugumye
occiput *Back of the head.*	agakomokomo
occlusion *A pathway that is blocked or obstructed.*	kuzibira
occupational therapist *A clinician who specializes in rehabilitation of persons with upper extremity disorders.*	ujejwe kunonora imitsi ku kazi
ocular paralysis. *Paralysis of intraocular and extraocular muscles.*	umusonga muryinyo
odiferous *Having an unpleasant or distinctive smell.*	umunuko
odontalgia *Tooth pain.*	gukongatara kwamaso
odor *A smell that is given off someone or something.*	ubumote
odynophagia *Pain associated with swallowing.*	kubabara mukukira
offspring *One's children. (child)*	uruvyaro
ointment *A petroleum jelly based topical medication.*	amafata y'ukwisiga
old age *A relative term for the period of advanced years.*	ubusaza
older *Being around more than compared with another.*	gusaza
olecranon *The bony protrusion at the proximal ulna at the elbow.*	inkokora
olfactory *Referring to the sense of smell.*	kumotera
oligodactyly *Presence of fewer than 5 digits on a hand or foot.*	kugira intoke nke
oligohydramnios *Inadequate amount of amniotic fluid.*	kugira amazi make mugitereko, kumugore yibungenze
oligomenorrhea *Infrequent menstruation or low volume menstrual flow.*	kuja mukwezi gake
oligotrophia or hypotrichosis *Less than normal amount of head/body hair.*	kugira umushatsi muke
oliguria *Abnormally low urine output.*	Gusoba duke
omentum *A peritoneal fold passing from the stomach to another abdominal organ.*	ikinure
omphalitis *Inflammation of the umbilicus.*	indwara y umukondo
on going *Continuing,*	uwuronderezi
oncologist *A physician specializing in the treatment of cancer.*	umuganga wa kanseri
onset *The beginning of an event.*	umuwanzo
onychia *Inflammation of the toenail or fingernail matrix.*	indwara yo kunzara
onychomycosis *Fungal disease of the toenails or fingernails.*	indwara yo kunzara
onychophagia *Habitually chewing on one's fingernails.*	Kurya-Guhekenya inzara zo ku ntoke
ooze, to *To slowly leak.*	kuwira wyuya
operation *A surgical procedure. (to operate)*	ukubaga (kubaga)

English	Kirundi
ophthalmia *Profound inflammation of the eye or its structures.*	indwara y amaso
ophthalmologist *A physician specializing in diseases of the eye.*	muganga w'amaso (muganga ubaga)
opium *An addictive drug derived from opium poppy; synthetic versions are used as analgesics.*	umuti wubububabare
optometrist *A person who practices optometry.*	muganga w'amaso
oral *Relating to the mouth.*	mukanwa
oral contraceptive *Tablet taken by mouth to prevent pregnancy.*	imiti yo kuringaniza uruvyaro
orally *By mouth. (verbally)*	mukanwa
oral medication *Medicine taken by mouth.*	imiti yo mu kanwa
orbit *The bony structure enclosing the eyeball.*	intoboro y'ijisho
orchialgia *Testicular pain.*	umusonga wo mw ivya
orchidectomy *Synonym of orchiectomy; removal of one or both testes.*	kubaga ivya
orchitis *Inflammation of one or both testes.*	indwara y amavya
orphan *A child without parents*	impfuvyi
oropharynx *The portion of the pharynx between the soft palate and the superior aspect of the epiglottis.*	mu magage
orthopedics *A surgical specialty concerned with treatment of skeletal problems.*	kunonosora ivyirwa vyo kubaga
orthopnea *The inability to breath comfortably except in the upright position.*	guhema nabi
osteomyelitis *Inflammation of the bone or bone marrow because of a microorganism.*	umegera w amagufa n imitsi
osteoporosis *Loss of bone substance because the osteoblasts fail to produce bone matrix.*	gusaza kwamagufa
osteotomy *Creation of a surgical opening in bone.*	kubaga igufa
otalgia *Ear pain.*	umusonga wo mu matwi
otitis externa *Inflammation of the middle ear*	indwara zo mu matwi
otitis *Inflammation of the ear. (otitis media or otitis externa)*	indwara y amatwi
otomycosis *Fungal infection of the ear.*	indwara y amatwi
outdated *Something that has passed the expiration date.*	guta igihe
ovary *One of a paired of female reproductive glands containing oocytes.*	agassaho kimbuto zumugore
overdose *An above normal dose of a medication.*	kurenza urugero rwumuti
overt *Not hidden.*	ikivugwa
overweight *To be above the normal body mass index (BMI).*	kugira ibiro
oviduct *The channel which an ovum passes from the ovary.*	uturingoti imbuto zicamwo
ovulation *The release of an ova from the ovary.*	kuja mubutinyanka
owing to *On account of.*	gukenerwa gu…
oxygen *A colorless, odorless gas with atomic number 8.*	umwuka, impwemu
pace *Consistent and continuous movement.*	intambwe
pachydermia *An abnormally thick skin.*	urukoba rwonze
pain *Physical suffering or discomfort.*	ububabare
painless *Not painful.*	kitababaza
palate *The roof of the mouth.*	uruhekenyero; amagage
palatoplegia *Paralysis of the palate.*	kutimba kwakamirampeke

English	Kirundi
pallidectomy *Surgical resection of all or part of the palate.*	kubaga akamirampeke
pallor *Unusually pale appearance.*	ihindagana
palm *The anterior aspect of the hand.*	ikiganza
palpate,to *The assessment of the body with the use of one's hands.*	gukorakora
palpebra, palpebrae *Eyelid, eyelids.*	ingohe
palpitation *Sensation of a forceful, rapid, irregular heartbeat present after exercise or with anxiety.(to have palpitations)*	ukudihagizwa (kudidagira)
palsy *Paralysis that is usually associated with tremors.*	kijugumira
pancreas *A gland that secretes digestive enzymes into the duodenum and insulin and glucagon into the blood.*	igitabiza
pancreatectomy *Surgical excision of part or all of the pancreas.*	kubaga irwagasha
pancreatitis *Inflammation of the pancreas.*	Inndwara y urwagasha
pandemic *When a disease is present over an entire region.*	indwara y'ikiza gikwiye hose
panic attack *Sudden, profound anxiety.*	indwara yo kugira ubwoba budasanzwe
pap smear *Microscopic exam of cells from a swab of the cervix.*	gusuzumisha urwinjiriro rw'igitereko
papule *A small, well-circumscribed elevation of the skin.*	agahere
paracentesis *A procedure involving aspiration of fluid from the abdominal cavity.*	kuvoma amazi munda
paralysis *Inability to move one or more extremities.*	aramugaye; ubumuga
paralyzed, to be *To not be able to move one or more extremities.*	kumugara
paranasal *Situated adjacent to the nose.*	hafi y amazuru
paranoia *To have delusional thoughts.*	w'urwinubwe rurenze urugero.
paraplegia *Paralysis of the lower extremities.*	ubukongatare
pararectal *Adjacent to the rectum.*	hafi yigisusu
parasite *An organism that lives on or within another organism without benefit to the latter.*	ikiremwa nyohabuzima
paresis *Incomplete paralysis.*	ugutimba nk'igiti
paresthesia *An abnormal sensation usually described as pins and needles.*	ibinyanya
parietal bone *The bone on either side of the vault of the cranium.*	intera y'umutwe
paronychia *Inflammation of the tissue bordering a fingernail*	igihute co murwara
parturition *The process of giving birth.*	ukuvytara
pass, flatus to *To release bowel gas from the anus.*	gusurira
passive *Not achieved through active effort.*	areze amaboko
patella *The bone situated in the anterior portion of the knee.*	pia ya mguu; iyitfu m'ivi
patellectomy *Surgical excision of the patella.*	kubaga ivi
pathogenesis *The course of a disease.*	insiguro y indwara
patient *The client being treated for a medical or surgical condition.*	umugwayi
patient, to be *To be unhurried.*	kwihangana
pediatrician *Physician who is a specialist in pediatrics.*	umuganga w'abana
pediculosis *Lice infestation.*	umurwayi

English	Kirundi
pelvic inflammatory disease *Generally a bacterial infection affecting a women with potential involvement of the uterus, fallopian tubes, ovaries and cervix.*	indwara yo mubihimba vy rondoka
pelvis *The boney structure connecting the spine with the legs.*	urukenyerero
pemphigus *A skin disorder with large bullous lesions.*	indwara y'amabavu
penis *Male genital organ used for the transfer of sperm and elimination of urine.*	imboro
perforation *Presence of a hole.*	ugutobora
pericardial tamponade *Decrease in systemic perfusion related to a collection of fluid in the pericardial space.*	indwara yumutima
pericarditis *Inflammation of the pericardium.*	indwarayumutima
pericardium *The structure enclosing the heart which contains a fibrous outer layer and serous inner layer.*	isaho y'umutima
perineal *Referring to the perineum.*	kugisusu
perinephric *Around the kidney.*	impande y amafyigo
perineum *The area between the anus and scrotum or anus and vulva.*	umwararo
peripheral *Referring to an outward part or surface.*	kwiherezo
peristalsis *The contractile action of the bowel.*	isunikwa ry'ivyinjijwe mu mara
peritoneum *The serous membrane covering the abdominal organs and lining the abdominal walls.*	isaho nkingiramara
peritonitis *Inflammation of the peritoneum.*	ubuvyimbe bw'isaho nkingiramara
peritonsillar abscess	igihuteco mukannwa
personality *Qualities that form a person's unique character.*	akaranga k ubuntu
perspiration from armpit (or bad body odor)	igikakwe
perspiration *The process of sweating.*	icuya
perspire heavily, to *To sweat more than one would normally.*	kubira icuya
pertussis *Synonym for whooping cough.*	inkorora y'akanira
pes cavus *Excessive height of the longitudinal arch of the foot.*	ubwami bwikirenge bunini
pes planus *Medical term for flat foot.*	ikirenge gifyase
Peyronie's disease *Curvature of the penis during an erection due to plaque.*	indwara ya Peyironi
phalanges *The long bones of the fingers or toes.*	ingingo
phantom limb pain *Pain sensed in an area where one has had an amputation as though the limb is still present.*	umusonga waho baciye igihimba
pharmacist *A professional who prepares and sells medicine through various systems, including governmental organizations like the Veterans Administration.*	umuhinga mu n'imiti
pharmacy *A business that sells prescription medication.*	iforomasiyo
pharyngitis *Inflammation of the pharynx.*	ukuvyimba imiriro
pharynx *The membranous cavity from the mouth to esophagus. (umio is sometimes used to describe esophagus at also the larynx)*	umuhogo
phlebotomy *The removal of blood for testing or as a therpeutic intervention.*	ubuhinga bwo kufata amaraso mu mitsi
phlegm *Sputum.*	igikororwa
phobia *An profound fear of something.*	ubwoba

English	Kirundi
photophobia *Abnormal sensitivity to light.*	gutinya umuco
physical exam *Examination of a client to assess their medical status.*	kwitfatisha ibipimo vyuzuye kwa muganga
physical therapist *Clinician who specializes in rehabilitation of persons with lower extremity disorders.*	muganga gorora abamugaye; abavunitse canke abahinyagaye
physical therapy *Treatment of disease by heat, massage and exercise as opposed to medications.*	kugirwa inama; imyimenyerezo
physician *Medical practitioner.*	umuganga
pia mater *The first layer of three covering the brain and spinal cord.*	igihimba c ubwonko
pill *A medicated tablet or capsule.*	umuti; ikinini
pillow *An encased fabric covering soft material used for a cushion.*	umusego
pink eye *Common term for acute contagious conjunctivitis.*	uburire
pinworm *Common term for Enterobius vermincularis; a nematode worm that is a parasite.*	inzoka yo umubiri
placenta *The vascular tissue that nourishes a fetus through an umbilical cord.*	kuragar'ingovi; ingovyi
placenta praevia *A condition in which the placenta covers the cervical os.*	ingovyi izibira umwana
placental abruption *Premature detachment of a normally situated placenta.*	ingovyi yahomotse
plantar *Referring to the bottom of the foot.*	mu kirenge
plantar wart *A viral epidermal growth on the bottom of the foot.*	umugera wo mukirenge
plaster cast *Use of gypsum impregnated gauze to immobilize fractured extremities.*	isima
plethora *An excess of something.*	ubwinshi
pleura *The serous membrane lining each lung.*	agapfukahaha
pleurisy *Inflammation of the pleura.*	igifuka
pneumocystis jiroveci pneumonia. *A pulmonary infection associated with AIDS. Formerly called pneumocystis carinii pneumonia*	indwara zivyuririzi
pneumonectomy *Surgical excision of all or part of a lung.*	kubaga ihaha
pneumonia *Inflammation of the lung due to an infection caused by a virus or bacterium.*	umusonga
pneumothorax *Abnormal presence of air between the lung and chest wall.*	indwara y iyinjira ry impemu mu mahaha
podiatrist *Physician, surgeon specializes in disorders of the feet.*	muganga w'ibirenge
poison *A substance that causes illness or death.*	uburozi
poliomyelitis *An infectious viral disease exhibited by constitutional symptoms that can lead to quadriplegia.*	ubukangwe
polydactyly *Congenital anomaly exhibited by more than 5 digits on the hands and/or feet.*	intoke nyinshi
polydipsia *Profound thirst.*	inyota nyinshi
polysialia *Abnormal increase in saliva.*	urukonda
polyuria *Abnormal increase in volume of urine excreted.*	kunyaragura

English	Kirundi
popliteal fossa *The hollow in the posterior aspect of the knee joint.*	muntege
port-wine mark *Also called nevus flammeus, it is a vascular anomaly characterized by purplish skin discoloration.*	indwara y ihinduka ryurukoba
positive *Indicating the presence of something.*	neza
post-term birth *An infant born after the normal length of pregnancy.*	kurenza iariki yokuvuka
posterior *Further back in position; opposite of anterior.*	co hanyuma
postictal *The period of time after a seizure.*	igihe cinyuma yibisahuzi
post-operative *Referring to the time after an operation.*	c'inyuma y'ibagwa
post-partum depression *Depressed mood occurring after childbirth.*	indwara yo mu mutwe ikurikira kwibaruka
post-partum psychosis *A episode of abnormal thought or hallucinations following delivery.*	indwara yomumutwe yinyuma yo kwibaruka
postpone, to *To delay.*	kuhindura amatariki
post-traumatic stress syndrome (PTSD)	inkurikizi zo guhahamuka; indwara nyakuri
potency *Strength or power.*	inguvu
powder *Fine dry particles.*	ipuderi
preauricular *Anterior to the ear.*	imbere y ugutwi
pre-conception health *The health habits, medications and nutritional status of a woman before becoming pregnant.t*	amagara y'umukenyezi imbere yuko asama
pregnancy *The period of being pregnant.*	inda
pregnant, to be	gusama inda; kuremerwa
pregnancy test, to get a	gupimisha imbanyi
pregnant woman	umugore yibungenze
premature *Occurring earlier than expected.*	kitaragera
premenstrual *Occurring prior to the onset of menstruation.*	c'imbere y'ubutinyanka
premenstrual syndrome *A cluster of emotional, behavioral, and physical symptoms that occur in the premenstrual phase of the menstrual cycle and resolve with the onset of menstruation.*	imisonga yo mukwezi
prenatal *Referring to the time prior to birth.*	c'imbere yo kwibaruka
prenatal care *The medical care received after becoming pregnant and before childbirth.*	genda kwa muganga kaurikirane ivyerekeye amagara yawe n'amagara y'ibondo utwaye
prepuce of clitoris *The external skin fold of the labia minora which forms a cap over the clitoris.*	inankunkuma
presbyopia *Farsightedness associated with aging.*	indwara y'amaso iterwa n'ubusaza
prescription *The action of prescribing a medication or treatment.*	umuti wanditswe n'umuganga
presenting symptom *The initial subjective complaint that initiated a visit.*	intanguro y indwara
pressure dressing *A dressing used for compression to reduce bleeding.*	ipansuma yo guhagarika kuva amaraso
pressure ulcer *Loss in skin integrity due to a portion of the body being in the same position for too long and possibly other factors.*	igikomere co kuremerwa

97

English	Kirundi
prevent, to *To stave off or hinder.*	kubuza
priapism *A painful and abnormally prolonged erection.*	imisonga iza mumwanya wo gushukwa
primipara *A woman giving birth for the first time.*	uruvyaro rwambere
problem *Difficulty or complaint.*	ingorane
proctectomy *Surgical excision of the rectum.*	kubagwa mu gisusu
proctitis *Inflammation of the rectum.*	indwara yo mugisusu
prognosis *The likely course of a disease.*	ivyitezwe mu bipimo vy'indwara
progressive *Developing gradually.*	kiba intabwe ku yindi
prolapse of the rectum *Terminal portion of the rectum comes through the anus.*	uracuye ku'mugongo
prolapse of the umbilical cord *Refers to the umbilical cord protruding from the cervix during active labor.*	isohoka ryuruzogi imbanyi itaravuka
prolapse of the uterus *Eversion of the uterus through the vagina.*	indwara yigitereko gisohokera mu gisundi
prolonged rupture of the membranes *Rupture of the membranes more than 24 hours before delivery.*	amazi yumwana aseseka umwanya muremure
pronation *Turning posteriorly. When the hand is pronated, it is turned medially until the palm is facing posteriorly (when the body was initially in the anatomic position).*	guhindukiriza inyuma
prone *Lying with the abdomen and face downward.*	kwubika inda
prophylaxis *That which is done to prevent disease.*	ukuzitira utaronerwa
prostate *A gland found in men that surrounds the neck of the urethra and bladder.*	prostate (ari ko gasabo gakikije umuyoboro usohora inkari ku mugabo).
prostatectomy *Surgical excision of the prostate.*	kubaga prostate
prostatitis *Inflammation of the prostate gland.*	uruvya
prosthesis *An artificial body part. (above the knee) [below the knee]*	igihimba nterano cokwivi
prostitute *A person who exchanges goods or services for sex.*	indaya
prostration *Profound exhaustion.*	gutubwenge
protein *A class of nitrogenous organic compound.*	inyubakaambubiri
proteinuria *The presence of protein in the urine.*	umukoyo urimwo proteini
provoke, to *To evoke or elicit.*	kwandurutsa
proximal *Situated closer to the center of the body (opposed to that which is farther away, as in distal).*	hejuru
pruritus *A general term for conditions exhibited by itching.*	kwiyahaza
psychiatrist *A doctor who treats persons with problems of the human mind and emotions and can prescribe medication.*	umuganga bw'indwara zo mu mutwe
psychologist *Clinician with a doctorate degree who specializes in treatment of mental disorders without the use of medications.*	muganga ujejwe ingorane zo
psychology *The study of the human mind and emotions.*	ubuhinga bw'ukwiyumvira n'inyifato
psychosis *A profound mental disorder that can include delusions and hallucinations.*	indwara yo guta umutwe
ptosis *Drooping of the upper eyelid usually due to paralysis of the third cranial nerve.*	ugutimba kwingohe

puberty *The time when adolescents become capable of sexual reproduction.* — ibigero

pubic hair *Hair present in the perineal area.* — inzya

pubis *The anterior inferior part of the hip bone on each side that articulates at the pubic symphysis.* — intantu

puffiness *Having a soft, swollen area.* — umubiri wavyimvye

pull, to *To exert force on something.* — gukweka

pulmonary edema *Characterized by abnormal fluid buildup in the lungs.* — indwara yo kwuzura amazi mumahaha

pulmonary embolism *A sudden blockage of a lung artery frequently emanating from a blood clot in one's leg.* — indwara yo kubura amaraso mumahaha

pulmonary *Referring to the lungs.* — kinanye n'amahaha

pulp *The tissue filling the root canals of a tooth.* — umuzi wiryinyo

pulpitis *Dental pulp inflammation.* — indwarayo mumuzi windyinyo

pulse *The rhythmic throbbing of arteries felt at major vessels.* — indihagizi

pupil *The opening at the center of the iris.* — imbonero

purulent *Referring to pus.* — kuva amashira

pus *Thick yellow or green opaque liquid as seen with infection.* — amashira

pyorrhea *Emission of pus.* — gusohora amashira

pyrexia *Fever.* — umuriro

pyrosis *Synonym for heartburn.* — ikirungurira

pyuria *Presence of purulent material in the urine.* — gusoba amashira

quadriceps *The anterior thigh muscle composed of four muscles.* — imitsi yo kwitako

quadriplegia *Paralysis of all four extremities.* — gutimba umubiri wose

qualify *To become eligible by fulfilling a necessary standard.* — gushoboza

quarantine *A place of isolation for infectious persons until it can be certain it is safe to let them mingle.* — ugukumira

quickening *Signs of life noted by a mother as the fetus moves.* — kinyaruka

quiescent *A time of inactivity.* — gihwekereye

quiet,to be *Making little or no noise.* — kunuma

quinsy *Peritonsillar inflammation or abscess.* — igihute co mumagage

rabies *An infectious viral disease transmitted through the bite of a mammal. Symptoms include hydrophobia, pharyngeal spasms and hyperactivity.* — indwara iterwa no kurumwa n'inyamaswa

radial *Referring to the radius.* — radial> igihande co hejuru yukoboko

radiation *1. The emission of energy in the form of electromagnetic waves. 2. Divergence from a common point.* — ikibengebenge (1)

rage *Uncontrollable anger.* — ibisazi

raise, to *To lift or bring up.* — gusokora

rape,to *Forced sexual relations.* — guterura

Rapid Eye Movement *The movement of a person's eyes during this period of sleep.* — guhindukiza amaso cane

rash *Exanthema or urticaria.* — amahere

rat *A rodent that looks like a large mouse.* — imbeba

rat bite fever *As the name implies, it is a condition exhibited by fever, nausea and skin erythema after one is bitten by a rat.* — indwara yo gushuha

English	Kirundi
reaction *A response to an action.*	inyishu
rebound *A term used to describe a type of tenderness found with peritonitis.*	gusasatwa munda
recollection *Memory.*	ukwibuka
recover,to *(from a serious ailment)*	kurokoka
recover from a grave illness, to	gukira
rectal digital examination *Use of a gloved finger to assess the rectal vault.*	gupima mugisusu nurutoki
rectal *Referring to the rectum.*	mugisusu
rectum *The terminal portion of the digestive tract extending from the distal sigmoid to the anus.*	umurongoro
recurrent fever *Repeated fever from an unknown cause.*	kimputo
reduction *Return of a dislocated joint or fractured bone to its proper position.*	gukosora amagufa yatiriganye
regardless of *Without consideration of.*	utwininga
regurgitation *1. Backflow of blood in the heart. 2. Movement of gastric contents into the mouth.*	gusubiramwo
relapsing fever *A recurrent bacterial infection, with fever, caused by Spirochetes.*	kimputo
related to *Causally connected.*	bijanye na.
relation *1. A person who has a blood or marriage connection.*	incuti
reliable *Trustworthy.*	kwizera
relief *Alleviation from pain or discomfort.*	ukworoherwa
relieve, to (pain) *To make less severe.*	gutezura
REM (rapid eye movement) sleep *This period of sleep is associated with irregular respirations and heart rate, involuntary movements and dreaming.*	guhindukiza amaso cane mwitiro
remission *A decrease in severity or a temporary resolution.*	gukira bukebuke
remove,to *The act of removing something.*	gukura
renal failure *Diminution of kidney function.*	indwara yamafyigo
resection *The removal of tissue.*	ugukura
respirator *A device used to artificially ventilate a patient.*	icuma gitanga umwuka
respiratory arrest *Cessation of breathing.*	guhagarika guhema
respiratory rate *The number of breaths per minute.*	incuro umuntu ahema kumunota
rest *Relaxation or respite.*	ikiruhuko
restless, to be *Wriggle or squirm. Extreme restlessness, tossing around in bed.*	kuruhukira cane mugitanda
retching *Spasm of the stomach without presence of gastric material.*	kuribwa mumushishito
retractor *A device for pulling back tissue during surgery.*	icuma gitandukanya inyama mukubaga
retrograde *Referring to backward movement.*	gusubira inyuma
rheumatic pain *Pain related to rheumatoid arthritis.*	imisonga ya rimatizime
rheumatism *Any condition exhibited by inflammation and pain in the joints and muscles.*	rimatizime
rhinitis *A viral infection or allergic reaction exhibited by nasal mucosal inflammation.*	indwara yo mumazuru

English	Kirundi
rhinoplasty *Plastic surgery performed on the nose.*	kubaga mumazuru
rhinorrhea *Abundant nasal mucosal drainage.*	ibicurane; ibiseru
rhythm *The pattern or cadence.*	urugero
rib *One of a series of curved paired boney articulations protecting the thorax.*	urubavu
rickets *A condition exhibited by softening and bowing of the long bones; caused by Vitamin D deficiency.*	umuwango
Rift valley fever *A human febrile illness that is an endemic disease in sheep, transmitted by mosquitos and direct contact and caused by a virus of the family Bunyaviridae.*	indwara yubushuhe
right *Correct, accurate (adjective)*	c'ukuri
right *Justice or fairness.(noun)*	agateka
right *When referring to the right hand or side.*	uburyo
right *Sure, agreed, OK (adverb)*	nuko; niko
right-handed *Having a preference to use the right hand.*	gukoresha ukuryo cane
rigor mortis *The normal stiffening of the muscles and joints that occurs a few hours after death.*	gutimba kwumupfu
ringing in the ears *Common term for tinnitus.*	kwiyagaza mumatwi
risus sardonicus *A spasm of the facial muscles causing what appears to be a smile on one's face.*	indwara y imitsi yo mumaso
rodent *A gnawing mammal that includes rats and mice.*	imbeba
rotation *Movement around an axis.*	kuyunguruka
rotator cuff *The structure around the capsule of the shoulder joint formed by the infraspinatus, supraspinatus, teres minor and subscapularis muscles.*	inyama yo mwiteraniro ryurutugu
rubella *Also called German measles, it is characterized by a rash, fever, headache.*	ibihara
rude *Ill-mannered.*	umuhurudutsi
running suture *A method of sewing a wound in which there is a knot at each end and continuous otherwise.*	gushona
rupia *A sign of tertiary syphilis in which there are bullae or vesicles formed on the skin that erupt and form crusts.*	ikimenyeco cindwara ya mburugu
rupture *An instance of bursting suddenly.*	gupasuka
ruptured membranes *Signal of onset of labor*	agakoko kagurutse, or amazi yasesetse
sacrum *The bone formed by five fused vertebrae that is situated between the two hip bones.*	ikigongogongo
sadness *The state of being sad.*	akabonge
saline *A solution of sodium chloride.*	umunyu
saliva *The watery liquid secreted by the salivary glands.*	amate
salivation *The process of secreting saliva.*	agakiza
salpingitis *Inflammation of the fallopian tubes.*	indwara yo muduheha dutwara imbuto mugitereko kumugore

English	Kirundi
salt *Typically referring to sodium chloride.*	umunyu
sandfly fever *A febrile illness transmitted by a sandfly, from the genus Phlebotomus, and found in the Mediterranean.*	Indwara y ubushuhe
sanitary napkin *Cloth or synthetic material used to absorb menstrual blood.*	agaswime
saponify,to *The creation of soap from oil using an alkali.*	guhingura isabuni
saturation *An amount, expressed in a percentage, that expresses the degree something is absorbed versus the maximal absorption possible.*	kwuzurana
saw *A hand or power-driven tool used for cutting.*	umusumeno
scabies *A skin condition exhibited by intense pruritus and a macular rash commonly in the perineal and interdigital spaces.*	ihere
scald *A burn injury from extremely hot water.*	igisebe kivuye kuguturirwa namazi ashushe cane
scale *A device to check a person's weight.*	umunzane
scalp *The skin covering the head except for the face.*	urukoba rwo kumushatsi
scalpel *A knife used during surgery for incision of skin and tissue.*	imbugita yo kubaga
scapula *Medical term for the shoulder blade.*	urushi w'ukuwoko
scar *The fibrotic tissue that forms at the site of a wound.*	inkovu
scarlet fever *A condition caused by streptococci that is exhibited by fever and a bright red (scarlet) rash.*	indwara yubushuhe
scatter *The degree to which repeated measurements differ.*	gusanza
scheme *A program or plan.*	umurongo ngenderwako
schistosomiasis *A condition, sometimes known as bilharzia, which involves infestation with flukes of the genus Schistosoma.*	birariziyoze
schizophrenia *A chronic mental condition exhibited by delusions, hallucinations, and faulty perception.*	indwara yo mumutwe
shower chair *A seating device one sits on while showering.*	intebe bicarako mu koga
scissors *A cutting instrument with two blades, joined at the middle.*	umukasi wo kubaga
sclera *The white outer covering of the eyeball.*	ikidzjicyo cyera
scleritis *Inflammation of the eyeball.*	indwara y amaso
sclerotomy *Surgical incision of the sclera.*	kubaga mumaso
scoliosis *A lateral curvature of the spine.*	indwara yumugongo
scrape *An injury caused by having a body part rubbed against a rough surface.*	ubuharura
scratch *A long, narrow superficial wound.*	umukwabu
screening *An evaluation as part of a methodical study.*	gupima
scrotum *The sac which contains the testes.*	umuruga
scurvy *A disease of vitamin C deficiency exhibited by bleeding gums.*	kuva amaraso mu kanwa, indwara yibura rya vitamine c
secretion *The discharge of substances from cells or glands.*	amazi ava mumubiri
sedative *A medication used to facilitate sleep or calm a person.*	gusinziriza

English	Kirundi
see the doctor, to	kubonana na muganga
seizure *An episode of tonic/clonic movement noted in epilepsy.*	ibisahuzi
semen	intanga
semen analysis *Evaluation of semen used as part of a fertility workup.*	gupima intanga
seminoma *A malignant tumor of the testis.*	ikivyimba co mumavya
sensation *A perception when one is touched.*	kwumva uwugukozeko
sepsis *A condition exhibited by overwhelming inflammation due to infection.*	kugira mikorobe nyinshi mu maraso
septicemia *A systemic disease in which microorganisms or their toxins are in the blood stream.*	indwara yamaraso, afise mikorobe nyinshi
septum *A wall separating two chambers, the nasal septum for example.*	igihimba co muzuru
sequela *A medical problem related to an initial injury or disease.(late sequelae)*	inkurikizi
sequestrum *Necrotic bone present in an injured or diseased bone.*	igufa ryaboze
serial *In a series.*	mu migwi
serum *The fluid that isolates out when blood coagulates.*	serumu
severe *Intense or very great.*	gikaze
sex *Gender.*	igitsina
sexual intercourse *The act of copulation.*	guhuza ibitsina
sexually transmitted disease (STD) *A condition one obtains from another during sexual relations.*	indwara zo mu bihimba vy'irondoka
shake, to *To tremble uncontrollably.*	guceka
sharp (pain) *When describing pain, a piercing sensation.*	ubwoko bwumusonga
sheath *A covering.*	urwubati
sheet (bed) *A rectangular fabric covering a bed.*	ishuka
shellfish *An aquatic shelled crustacean or mollusk.*	ikinyamwonga
shin *Refers to the anterior tibial region.*	umurundi
shingles *A reactivation of herpes zoster.*	umugera wa herpes
shiver *A trembling. (to shiver)*	umushitsi (kuja mu gashitsi)
shock *Surprise or astonishment. (startled)*	akababaro
shoe *Article of clothing worn on each foot.*	ikirato
shortening *Notable for having a shorter length.*	igabanuka
shoulder *The joint were the scapula joins the clavicle and humerus. (right shoulder, left shoulder)*	urutuga
shunt *An alternate path for blood or fluid.*	inzira igomorora amaraso canke amazi yo mumubiri
sibling *A brother or sister. (younger sibling)*	umuvukanyi
sick child	uruzingo
sick person	umurwayi
sick, to be	kuwara
sickness *Illness or a state of disease.*	indwara
side *A position medial or lateral to center.*	imbavu
side effect *An expected but unwanted effect of a medication.*	inkurikizi
sigh,to *A long deep exhalation that expresses an emotion, as in relief.*	kuniha

103

English	Kirundi
silent,to be *Absence of noise or no indication of something.*	guhora
simultaneous *Occurring at the same time.*	bibera icarimwe
single woman (single man) *Not married.*	inkumi (umusore)
single *Only one.*	kimwe
sinusitis *Inflammation of the sinuses.*	amasinizite
sip, to *To slowly take small drinks of a fluid.*	gusoma dukeya
sit, to	kwicara
site *Location.*	ikibanza
size *The dimensions of something.*	ubunini
skeleton *Internal bony framework.*	amagufa
skin *Flesh.*	urusato; umuhiro
skin disease that causes red spots,to have	guturika
skin fold *An overlapping of skin formed by subcutaneous tissue.*	umuhiro y'amatako
skin rash *Dermal exanthema.*	amahere
sleep *A nap or a snooze. (deep sleep)*	itori
sleep,to *The act of sleeping*	gusinzira
sleep apnea *Episodic apnea during sleep that is exhibited by daytime symptoms of fatigue, difficulty concentrating and sleepiness.*	indwara yo kubura impwemu mwijoro
sleeping sickness *Also called Trypanosomiasis, this disease is caused by a parasitic protozoa and transmitted by the tsetse fly.*	uruwe
slight *Minor or small.*	buhoro
slow *Unhurried.*	buhoro
sludge *A viscous fluid.*	birenduka
slurring *Indistinct yet comprehensible speech.*	kututisha ururimi
smallpox *Variola.*	akaranda; ibihara
smegma *A thick curdled secretion found around the clitoris and the prepuce.*	amazi yo mubihimba vyirondoka
smile, to *To spread the mouth with the edges upright.*	kunyinyura
smoke, to *To inhale on a cigarette.*	kunywa itabi
snake (snake venom)	inzoka; ikiyoka
sneeze, to *To suddenly expel air from the nose and mouth because of nasal irritation. (a sneeze)*	kwasamura
sniff,to *Short, rapid nasal inhalation. (or to smell)*	guhema itama rimwe
snore, to *To snore or grunt while breathing during sleep. (a snore)*	gufuhagira
snuff *Chewing tobacco.*	kukwega itabi
soap *A compound made with fats/oils and an alkali; it is used for washing.*	isabuni
sob, to *To cry uncontrollably.*	kubogoza
socks *Worn on the feet before one puts on shoes.*	amashesheti
sodium chloride *A colorless, crystalline compound; also table salt.*	umunya
soft,to be *Easy to mold or compress.*	kworoha
sole of foot *Common term for plantar aspect of the foot.*	mubworo bwikirenge
somnambulism *Sleepwalking.*	indwara yo kugendagenda umuntu asinziriye

English	Kirundi
somnolence *Drowsiness.*	kwayura
sorcery *Black magic or voodoo.*	Kuragura
sore throat *Common term for pharyngitis.*	ukuvyimba imiriro
sore *An ulcer or lesion.*	igikomere
sound *Vibrations that travel through air and are heard when reaching the ears.*	ijwi
sour *An acid or bitter taste.*	urubu
span *A distance between two objects.*	urugero
spasm,to have a *An involuntary contraction of muscles.*	gusamba
speak,to *To talk.*	kuvuga
specific *Clearly defined.*	nyayo
speech *Oral articulation.*	imvugo
speech therapist *A person trained to assist people with speech and language disorders.*	ujejwe ingorane zijanye no
sperm *Short term for spermatozoon.*	intanga
spermatogenesis *The production of spermatozoa.*	ihingurwa ry intanga
spermicide *A substance capable of killing sperm.*	umuti wo kwica intanga
sphygmomanometer *Device for measuring blood pressure.*	akuma ko gupima umurindi wamaraso
spider	igitangurirwa
spinal cord abscess *A localized collection of purulent material in or adjacent to the spinal cord.*	igihute co mumugongo
spinal cord *The bundle of nerves that with the brain comprise the central nervous system.*	imitsi yo mumugongo
spine *The spinal column or a thorny protrusion.*	uruti rw'umugongo
spit *A term used to describe saliva that is ejected from the mouth.*	amate
spit,to *To expectorate or expel saliva from the mouth.*	gucira amate
spleen *The visceral organ that is involved with production and removal of blood cells.*	urwakashaya
splenectomy *Surgical excision of the spleen.*	kubaga urusina
splenomegaly *An abnormally enlarged spleen.*	kuvimba urwagashya
splint *A rigid support used to immobilize and extremity.*	icyungisho
sponge *Sterile fabric used to soak up fluid during surgery.*	agatambara ko guhanagura amaraso bariko barabaga
spontaneous *Occurring without provocation.*	kwizana
sprain, to have a *A joint injury without fracture.*	kuhunyayara
sputum *A mixture of respiratory tract secretions and saliva.*	igikororwa
squeeze, to *To apply pressure.*	gukanya
squint, to *To look at something with the eyes partially closed.*	guhunyereza
stab wound *An injury occurring with a sharp object.*	igikomere kiregeye
stabbing pain *A sharp piercing quality to pain.*	umusonga ushinga nkicumu
stagger, to *To walk in an unsteady fashion.*	guhushagirika
stamina *Ability to maintain physical or mental exertion for a long period.*	kwihagararako, 2. kurinda 3. kugira Ishaka (depends on the context)
stammer,to *The impulse to repeat the first letter of words and involuntary pauses while speaking.*	kugigimiza

English	Kirundi
stand, to *To stop or to be upright*	guhagarara
standing *Position or status.*	ishimikiro
starvation *Death related to starvation.*	isari
stasis *Lack of movement.*	kutanyeganyega
steatopyga *Excessive accumulation of fat in the buttocks.*	kuhinika
steatorrhea *Excrement with an abnormally high fat content.*	umusarani uvanze n amavuta
stenosis *Narrowing of an orifice.*	kwiyugara
stereognosis *The ability to identify an object by touch.*	ubushobozi bwo kwumva inkintu ugikozeko
sterile *1. Infertile 2. Refers to equipment that is free of contamination.*	kugumbaha (1)
sternum *Commonly called the breast bone, it consists of the corpus, manubrium and xiphoid process.*	inkoro; igufa ry'ikikaraza
stethoscope *Instrument used to listen to the heart and lungs.*	icuma gipima itera ry'umutima
stiff neck *Not easy to bend the neck without referring to a cause.*	urukebu
stillborn *Refers to a newborn that died in utero.*	umwana arafuye mu'nda
sting *A small puncture as in a bee sting.*	umugera
stink,to *To have a foul odor.*	kunuka
stitch *Common term for a sharp pain under the breast.*	ikishya
stomach *Organ of digestion between the esophagus and small bowel.*	inda; umushishito
stomach contents, undigested	amanyezi
stomach cramps *Sensation of muscle contraction in the epigastric area.*	inda haratotera
stomach ulcer *Gastric ulcer.*	iriseri yumushishito
stool *Feces, excrement.*	amavyi; umwanda mukuru; uho kwituma
stool, watery with mucous	umusarani, amazi avanze nibirenduka
strain,to *As in a muscle strain.*	gukashuka
strain, knee *Knee pain severe enough to prevent one from walking.*	umukerecu
strength *Force, might or vigor.*	inkomezi
stress *Strain or pressure.*	agahinda
stretcher *A device used to carry a patient in the supine position.*	igitebo
stretcher used to carry a corpse	ikigagara
stridor *An abnormal, high-pitched, musical sound caused by an obstruction in the larynx or stenosis of the vocal cords.*	guhema nabi
stroke *Common term for cerebrovascular accident.*	n'indwara bukumbi y'ubwonko
strong,to be *Having the power to move heavy objects.*	gukomera
stump *Term used to designate what remains of an amputated extremity.*	igihimba gisigaye
stupor *A reduced level of consciousness.*	ukuraba
stutter,to *Involuntary repetition of the first consonant.*	kugigimiza
sty *Also called hordeolum externum, it is inflammation of the sebaceous gland of an eyelash.*	uruhongore rw'ingurube
subarachnoid *The layer of the brain covering between the arachnoid and pia mater.*	igihimba cubwonko

English	Kirundi
subdural *The area between the dura mater and the arachnoid membrane.*	ihigimba cumbwonko
sublingual *Situated under the tongue.*	munsi yururimi
submaxillary *Situated below the maxilla.*	munsi yimisaya
subungual *Under a fingernail or toenail.*	munsi yurwara
suck, to *As in, to suction fluid.*	kununuza
suckle, to *An infant taking to his mother's nipple.*	kwonka
suffer, to *To be affected by an illness or sickness.*	kubabara
suffocation *To die from a lack of air or inability to breathe.*	ukubura ihemero
sugar *A sweet crystalline substance made from a plant such as sugar cane.*	isukari
suicide *To kill oneself intentionally.*	ubwiyahuzi
superior *In a position above something else.*	hejuru
supine *Flat on one's back.*	uruti rwumugongo
supplies *Stock or reserves.*	integabiza
suppository *A delivery system for medication placed in an orifice.*	ikinini co mugisusu
suppuration *Formation of purulent material.*	kuva amashira
surgeon *A physician who performs surgery.*	umuganga abaga
surname *One's given "last" name that generally changes for women upon marriage to that of the man's surname.*	inzina ry'umuryango
sustain, to *To keep or maintain.*	kugumya
suture *Thread used for sewing together a wound.*	urunyuzi
swab *An absorbent material used for cleaning wounds or applying ointment.*	umuti wibikomere
swallow, to *To cause something to pass down the esophagus.*	kumira
sweat *Moisture exuded through the pores of the skin.*	icuya
sweat, to *The action of releasing moisture through pores of the skin.*	kubira icuya
swelling *An abnormal enlarged from fluid collection.*	ibutumbi
swell, to	kuvyimba
swollen (distended) abdomen	kuvyimba inda
symmetry *Being equally bilaterally.*	gusa, or kungana
symptom *A physical feature that is characteristic of disease.*	ikimenyetso c'indwara
syncope *Sudden loss of consciousness.*	ikifukunyi
synovial fluid *The fluid that surrounds, for example, the knee within a capsule.*	amavuta yo mumavi
syphilis *A infectious disease caused by Treponema pallidum that causes a painless penile ulcer in the primary stage but can lead to irreversible brain damage in the untreated tertiary stage.*	agashangara; isofisi
syringe *A device used for administering medication through various routes.*	urushinge
syrup *A thick sweet liquid.*	umuti wo kunywa
systolic *Referring to systole or that which occurs during systole.*	igipimo co hejuru cumurindi wamaraso
tablespoon *An eating utensil that holds 15milliliters of fluid.*	akayiko gato
tablet *A small disk of a compressed solid substance.*	umuti
tachycardia *Heart rate higher than physiologic normal.*	gusimbagurika umutima

English	Kirundi
tachypnea *Breathing faster than normal.*	guhezagirika
take medication, to	gufata umuti
talipes equinovaro *Medical term for what is commonly known as club foot.*	ubugaru
talus *The most superior tarsal bone that articulates with the tibia.*	idzjicyo ry'ikirenge
tape measure *A long length of tape, marked at intervals for measuring.*	imetero yo gupima
tapeworm *A parasitic, intestinal flatworm.*	igikangaga
tarantula *A large hairy spider found mainly in the tropics.*	igitangurirwa kinini
target *An objective towards which efforts are directed.*	intumbero
taste,to *Sensation of flavor perceived in one's mouth.*	kwumviriza
tattoo *A design made by inserting indelible ink into the skin.*	kwiraba (verb), imirabu (noun)
tear *As in a vaginal tear after childbirth.*	amarira
tears *Fluid expelled from the eyes during crying.*	amasozi
teaspoon *A measure instrument that holds 5 milliliters of fluid.*	ikiyiko kinini
teeth, front *The two maxillary teeth most anterior in the mouth.*	ishinyo
temperature *The degree of internal heat in a person's body.*	ubushuhe
temple *The temporal fossa superior to the zygomatic arch.*	umusaya
tendinitis *Inflammation of a tendon.*	indwara yimitsi (in kirundi, the tem imitsi has several meaning from different uses. It can be Vessels, Muscles, or tendons)
tendon *Fibrous tissue that connects muscle to bone.*	umurya
tepid *Lukewarm.*	akazuyazi
terminal illness *A disease with no viable treatment with death being inevitable.*	indwara idakira
testicle *One of a pair of organs in the male scrotum that produces sperm.*	itengatwa
testicular torsion *Rotation of the spermatic cord resulting in testicular ischemia.*	indwara yihotorwa ryivya
tetanus *A condition caused by Clostridium tetani which produces spasm and rigidity of voluntary muscles.*	tetanosi
thermometer *A device used to measure temperature.*	igipimabushuhe
thigh *The body region between the inguinal crease and knee.*	ikibero
thin *Lean or slender.*	kwonda
thin, to become *To lose a lot of weight.*	kwondesha
thirst *The desire to drink.*	inyota
thoracotomy *Surgical incision of the thorax.*	kubaga mugikiriza
thorax *The part of the body between the neck and abdomen.*	igikiriza
throat *The anterior aspect of the neck.*	umuhogo
throb, to *The beat with strong regular rhythm.*	gukubita kurugero rwo hejuru kandi rujanye
thrush *Candida albicans*	indwara y icuririzi ifata mu maso, mubihimba vyirondoka, mu marasocanke munzara
thumb *The first digit of each hand.*	urukumu

thyroid *A gland in the neck that secretes hormones regulating metabolism.* — agace gafatirako umwingo

thyroidectomy *Surgical resection of all or part of the thyroid.* — kubaga umwingo

tibia *The larger of two long bones in the lower leg.* — umugombero

tic *Periodic spasmodic facial muscle contractions.* — umusonga ufata imitsi yo mumaso

tick — inyondwi

tick-borne fever *A relapsing fever caused by a spirochete of the genus Borrelia.* — kimputo

tickle, to *To lightly touch a person to cause one to laugh.* — kudigadiga

tidal volume *The amount of air inspired with each breath. One can set a ventilator to deliver a preset number of milliliters of oxygenated air with each breath.* — impwemu zikoreshwa muguhema neza

tinea barbae *Ringworm on the face in the region a man shaves.* — ibifaranga

tinea capitis *Ringworm of the scalp, a fungal infection.* — indwara y'uburima

tinea corporis *Ringworm of the body, a fungal infection.* — ibisereka

tinea cruris *Ringworm in the inguinal region, a fungal infection.* — ibisereka

tinea pedis *Ringworm of the feet, a fungal infection.* — ibigatu

tinnitus *Medical term for ringing in the ears. It is associated with Meniere's syndrome among other conditions.* — kumva ingoma mumatwi

tired,to be *Fatigued.* — kuruha

toe *Any of the digits of of the feet.* — ino

toe, big *First digit of the foot.* — ino rinini

toenail *The nail at the tip/dorsal aspect of each toe.* — urwara

toilet *Device used during urination/defecation.* — akazu ka sugumwe

tongs *A medical device used for holding or grasping.* — icuma co gufata

tongue *The fleshy muscular organ of the mouth.* — ururimi

tonsils *A rounded mass of lymphoid tissue, most commonly referring to the pharyngeal tonsil.* — amagage

tonsillitis *Inflammation of the tonsils.* — arawaye mu muhogo

tooth *One of a set of hard, bony enamel coated structure in the jaw.* — iryinyo

toothache *Dental pain.* — ividzjekecyo

toothbrush *Handheld instrument used to clean one's teeth.* — Umujigiti; uburoso bwo koza amenyo

tooth, chipped *A tooth with a small piece broken off.* — virahongodotse

toothless *Edentulous.* — uwurozi

toothless person — ibihanga

toothpaste — umuti w'amenyo

torsion *Refers to twisting. Testicular torsion is the twisting of the spermatic cord that can lead to ischemia and gangrene of the testicle.* — guhotora

torso *The trunk of the body.* — intenga y'umuwiri

torticollis *A condition exhibited by the head being turned to one side continuously.* — kurwara izosi

touch,to *Tactile stimulation.* — gukorako

tourniquet *A device tied tightly around an extremity to diminish blood flow or blood loss.* — imbangwe

English	Kirundi
toxin *A poison of plant or animal origin.*	ubumara
trachea *The ringed canal between the pharynx and bronchi.*	igihogohogo
tracheitis *Inflammation of the trachea.*	indwara y igihogohogo
tracheostomy *Creation of a surgical opening in the trachea so a tube could be placed in the trachea.*	kubaga igihogohogo
trachoma *An infection of the cornea and conjunctiva caused by Chlamydia.*	indwara y amaso
tranquilizer *A medication used to diminish anxiety.*	umuti wo guhwamika
transdermal *Through the skin.*	murukoba
transfusion *Administration of blood products intravenously.*	gutera amaraso
transient ischemic attack *Cerebral ischemic changes resulting from transitory hypoperfusion.*	indwara y iyugagwa ry imitsi yamaraso yo mu bwonko
transplant,to *To move a body part from one location to another.*	gutera igihimba c'umubiri
trauma *A physical injury or emotional shock.*	akabonge
traumatic asphyxia *Cyanotic asphyxia due to trauma. Extravasation of blood into the skin and conjunctivae caused by a sudden increase in venous pressure from a crush injury.*	kubura impwemu
treat, to *Medical care one receives for illness or injury.*	kuvura
tremble from fever, to	gutetemera
tremble from fear, to	kugdegedwa
tremor *Involuntary contraction and relaxation of small muscle groups.*	gutetemera
trench mouth *Inflammation and ulceration of the gingivae.*	indwara y ibinyigishi
trendelenburg position *Position in bed in which the head is lower than the feet.*	kuryamira umugongo ucuramye
trichinosis *A disease caused by meat infected by Trichinella spiralis causing fever and gastrointestinal effects.*	indwara yo munda iterwa no kudya inyama yapfuye
triplets *Three infants born during one birth.*	ubushuri
trismus *Commonly called lockjaw, it is a spasm of the muscles supplied by the trigeminal nerve and is an early symptom of tetanus.*	kudadarara umunwa
trivial *Of little importance or value.*	bidakenewe
truss *A synthetic device for containing a hernia within the abdomen.*	icuma co gukosora indwara y umusipa
trypanosomiasis *A disease caused by a protozoa of the genus Trypanosoma that can cause sleeping sickness and Chagas' disease.*	ubusinziriza
tsetse fly *An insect that transmits the protozoa trypanosoma and can cause sleeping sickness.*	ikibugu
tuberculosis *Any infectious disease caused by Mycobacterium.*	igituntu
tuberosity *A protuberance. For instance the iliac tuberosity is a prominence on the surface of the ilium.*	ijisho bwigufa
tularemia *An infectious disease caused by Francisella tularensis. The symptoms range from mild constitutional complaints to septic shock.*	Indwara y ubushuhe ifatira kurukoba
tumor *A benign or malignant overgrowth of tissue.*	ikivyimba
twins *Two infants born at the same birthing.(identical twins)*	ihasi
two times *One action being done on two occasions.*	kabiri

English	Kirundi
tympanic membrane *The membrane between the external and middle ear.*	ingoma y ugutwi
tympanoplasty *Restoration of the tympanic membrane's continuity.*	Gukora ingoma y ugutwi
typhoid fever *A condition caused by ingestion of food or water containing salmonella typhi that is exhibited by fever and abdominal signs and symptoms.*	sutama; indwara y umwanda
typhus fever *A rickettsiae infection exhibited by rash, fever, headache and myalgia.*	tinfusi
ulcer *A concave wound caused by a break in the integrity of skin or mucous membrane. (duodenal ulcer)*	ikinutsi
ulna *The smaller bone in the forearm.*	igufa inini ry'inkokera
umbilical cord *The stalk between the placenta and the unborn infant.*	uruzogi
umbilical tape *Material used to tie off the umbilical cord prior to cutting it after the baby is born.*	akanyuzi ko kugenyera
umbilicus *The scar that denotes the end of the umbilical cord.*	umukondo
unconsciousness *Unable to respond to sensory stimuli.*	guta ubwenge
under; infra *Sometimes used when indicating a patient is "under treatment" for a condition (active treatment).*	munsi
undress *Take one's clothes off; disrobe.*	ambura; vanamo impuzu
underlying *Causative, unexposed, or fundamental.*	bikenewe
undulant fever *Wave-like variations in the fever, going from very high to normal and back again, as seen in Brucellosis.*	ubushuhe buza bukagenda
unexpected *Unforeseen.*	c'icubirizi
unknown *Uncertain or undisclosed.*	kitazwi
upper limb *Referring to either arm.*	ikizigira
upright *Vertical or standing.*	kimwenakimwe
ureter *The conduit between each kidney and the urinary bladder.*	inkaka
ureterectomy *Surgical resection of one or both ureters.*	kubaga uturingoti twumukoyo
ureteritis *Inflammation of the ureter.*	indwara yuturingoti twumukoyo
urethra *The canal connecting the urinary bladder with the outside of the body.*	uruhago
urethritis *Inflammation of the urethra.*	indwara yumuringoti nsozantaga
urethroplasty *Surgical repair of the urethra.*	gukosora umuringoti nsozantaga
urgency *Emergency or priority.*	vyihuta
urinal *Device used by men to void while in bed or sitting.*	isobero ryabagabo
urinalysis *Chemical and microscopic examination of the urine.*	gupima umukoyo
urinary bladder *The organ collecting urine from the ureters prior to discharge via the urethra.*	uruhago
urinary incontinence *Involuntary micturition.*	indwara yo kwisobako
urinary retention *Inadequately emptying the bladder.*	ikivyeyi
urinate,to	gusoba
urine *The fluid concentrated by the kidneys and expelled via the urethra.*	umwanda muto;inkari; amasobe
urticaria *A diffuse pruritic macular rash, caused by an allergy.*	urukushi
usual *Typical or normal.*	kimenyerewe

English	Kirundi
uterine bleeding *Bleeding that emanates from the uterus.*	kuva amaraso mu gitereko
uterus *The hollow organ in the female pelvis where a fertilized ovum embeds and grows.*	intanga; igitereko
uvula *A fleshy pendent at the back of the soft palate.*	amagage
uvulectomy *Excision of the uvula.*	gukata ikirimi
uvulitis *Inflammation of the uvula.*	indwara yikirimi
vaccination *The act of receiving a vaccine.*	ugucandaga
vaccine *A solution of attenuated microorganisms given to prevent or treat a disease.*	urucanco
vaccine certificate *A document that denotes what vaccines have been received by the holder.*	agatabu kicandarwa
vagina *The canal in a female that extends from the vulva to the cervix.*	igituba
vagina, opening of the	ikinogo
vaginal birth *Delivery of an infant through the vagina.*	kwibaruka biciye mu bihimba vy'irondoka
Valsalva's maneuver *A technique in which one attempts to exhale with the mouth and nose closed; this equalizes pressure in the ears.*	ubuhinga bwo guhemera mu matwi
varicella *A virus that causes chickenpox and shingles. Also called herpes zoster.*	agasama
varicocele *A cluster of varicose veins in the scrotum.*	ivyimba ry imitsi itwara amaraso mumavya
vascular *Referring to a blood vessel.*	imitisi yamaraso
vasoconstriction *The process of making the blood vessels smaller which increases blood pressure.*	iyugarwa ryimitsi yamaraso
vasodilatation *The process of making the blood vessels larger which decreases blood pressure.*	iyaguka ryimitsi itwara amaraso
vein *A vessel carrying blood back toward the heart.*	imudzi w'amaraso
venereal disease *A condition transmitted via sexual intercourse.*	indwara mpuzabitsina
venereal wart *Common term for condyloma acuminatum.*	indwara yo mubihimba vyirondoka
venom (snake) *A term used to describe the toxin injected via a bite or sting.*	ubumara
ventilation *The movement of air into the lungs; generally meant to suggest by an artificial process.*	ugutanga akayaga
ventral *Referring to the underside but in humans, a ventral hernia, for example, refers to an abdominal hernia.*	imbere,
ventricle *1. One of two chambers of the heart. 2. The four inter-connected cavities in the center of the brain.*	icumba
ventricular fibrillation *Chaotic and ineffective ventricular contractions.*	itera ryumutima mu rudubi
ventriculography *Roentgenography of the ventricles after administration of contrast media.*	imurikwa ry ivyumba vyumutima canke vyubwonko
verruca *A hyperplastic epidermal lesion, sometimes referred to as plantar wart.*	indwara y ukuvyimba mu kirenge
vertebra *A term for each bone surrounding the spine.*	igufa ryuruti rwumugongo
vertebral column *The cervical, thoracic and lumbar vertebrae.*	umurya w'umugongo
vertex *The crown of the head.*	intera y'umutwe

English	Kirundi
vertigo *A sensation of imbalance with many possible causes.*	impungenge
vesicle *A blister.*	utuhere
viable *Referring to a fetus that can survive childbirth.*	kubaho
viscous *Having a thick, sticky consistency.*	kirenduka
vision *State of being able to see.*	ukubona
vision, blurred *Haziness of the visual field.*	kubona ivyijiji
vitamin	imbumbamubiri
vitiligo *The appearance of non-pigmented white patches on otherwise normal skin; hair is usually white in the affected areas.*	ikihura
vocal cords *Paired folds of mucous membranes stretched across the larynx.*	izjwi
voice *The sound produced through the larynx and out the mouth.*	ijwi
voiding *The act of urinating.*	gukoyora
volunteer *A person who performs work without expecting compensation.*	umugiraneza
volvulus *Twisting of the bowel leading to obstruction and sometimes perforation.*	ihotorwa ryamara
vomit,to *The gastric contents that are expelled through the mouth.*	kuruka
vomit the mother's milk, to	kuboga
vulva *The external genitalia of the female.*	idururu
waddling gait *Walking in short steps in a swaying fashion.*	kunyoganyoga
waist *The part of the body between the ribs and the hips.*	urukenyerero
walk,to	kugenda
walker *A metal frame used to facilitate walking.*	igifasha umurwayi kugenda
ward *A section of a hospital where patients reside.*	icumba c abarwayi
wart *A flesh colored growth that is also called verruca.*	isununu
wart on clitoris	umugera wo ku gashino *(names of genital parts sound impolite, better to say . Umugera wo mubihimba vyirondoka)
wash in bed *Bed bath.*	kugereza umurwayi mu gitanda
wasp *Any one of a winged hymenopterous insects.*	ivubi
water *A colorless, odorless liquid.*	amazi
wax *Cerumen.*	ubukurugutwi
weak,to be *Feeble or deconditioned.*	kugira intege
weakness *Feebleness.*	ubumuga
weekly *That which occurs every seven days.*	ca buri ndwi
weep, to *To ooze fluid, such as from a wound.*	kuva amazi
weep, to *To shed tears.*	kurira
weigh, to	gupima
weight	uburiba
weight, to lose	kunamba
wet *Covered in moisture.*	gitose
wheal *A circumscribed urticarial lesion.*	igikomere c umuzingi
wheelchair *A wheeled device used for propulsion.*	intebe yo gusunika umugwayi

English	Kirundi
wheeze	uguhezera
wheeze,to	guhezera
whisper,to *Speech in a volume that is barely discernible.*	kwitonganya
whistle, to *To make a high pitch noise by forcing air through the lips.*	gufyfoza
whitlow *An abscess occurring on the palmar surface of the fingertips.*	utuhere
whooping cough *Pertussis*	inkorora y'akanira
widespread *Encompassing or spanning.*	cagutse
width *Side to side measurement.*	ubugari
wisdom tooth *Third molar.*	muzitsa
wise,to be *Possessing much knowledge.*	gukerebuka
withdrawal *The action of being without drugs or alcohol.*	ugusokora
withhold, to *To refuse to give something.*	kwima
World Health Organization (WHO)	Ishirahamwe Mpuzamakungu ry Amagara y Abantu.
worm *Any of long, slender, legless, soft-bodied invertebrates.*	inzoka
worry, to *To fret or have unease.*	gutamya
worsen, to *To deteriorate.*	kwunyuka
wound *A tissue injury of varying severity.*	ikinutsi
wrist *The articulation of the hand and radius/ulna.*	igikonjo
x-ray	iradiyo
xanthoma *A lipid deposition on the skin exhibited by an irregular yellow patch.*	umurabu wumuhondo uva kwigwirirana ryibinure kurukoba
xerophthalmia *A manifestation of Vitamin A deficiency exhibited by dryness of the cornea and conjunctiva.*	indwaa yo gukama amosozi
xerosis *Pathological dryness of the skin or mucous membranes.*	indwara yo kwuma urukoba
xiphoid process *The inferior segment of the sternum.*	akaziba kinda
yawn,to *Opening one's mouth and inhaling deeply due to sleepiness/boredom*	kwayura
yaws *A tropical disease characterized by ulcers on the extremities, caused by Treponema pertenue.*	ibinyoro
year *A time period that covers 365 days.*	umwaka
yearly *Occurring once each year.*	burimwaka
yeast *A unicellular fungus.*	umwambiro
yell, to *To speak in a loud tone.*	gutakana
yellow *A color between green and orange in the spectrum*	umuhondo
yellow fever *A viral, hemorrhagic fever transmitted by mosquitos.*	umugera wubushuhe uterwa nimibu (umupfube)
young *Having lived for a short period.*	mutoya
zero *No quantity.*	zero
zoology *The study of animals.*	icirwa cibikoko
zoonosis *An animal-born disease that can be transmitted to humans, such as rabies.*	indwara zibikoko zandukira abantu

Kirundi	English
-bisi	cold Having a sense of being cold.
-kazi (umuforomakazi)	female Feminine. (female nurse)
-rere	deep Having significant depth.
Aamtwi, Amatwi nimihogo	ENT Abbreviation for ears, nose and throat.
abangutse ibamfu	left-handed The preference of using the left hand for common tasks.
abasirikare bumubiri	lymphocyte A white blood cell produced by the lymph tissue.
abasoda bumubiri	blood cells A common term that does not differentiate between erythrocyte or leukocyte.
Abisirikare bumubiri	erythrocyte Called a red blood cell, it transports oxygen and carbon dioxide to and from the tissues.
adindye amaguru	lower extremity edema Interstitial edema of the legs.
afise amaso y'ubusaza	longsighted Synonym of hyperopia.
afise ubunebwe	indolent 1. Causing little pain. 2. Slow healing ulcer.
agace gafatirako umwingo	thyroid A gland in the neck that secretes hormones regulating metabolism.
agacupa	flask A narrow-necked container.
agahato	constriction Circumferential tightening
agahehera	coughing fit An episode of prolonged, forceful coughing.
agahehera (agahiri)	cold Viral upper respiratory tract infection.(cold in head)
agahere	papule A small, well-circumscribed elevation of the skin.
agaherera	catch a cold To come down with a viral upper respiratory tract infection.
agahinda	stress Strain or pressure.
agahitwe	diarrhea Increase in frequency and a loose consistency of the stools.
agahogohogo kaja mu mahaha	bronchus The major air channels that bifurcate from the distal trachea.
agakingirizo; udufuko	condom A covering for the penis or the vagina (female condom) used during sexual intercourse that is meant to reduce the chance of pregnancy or infection.
agakiza	salivation The process of secreting saliva.
agakoko kagurutse, or amazi yasesetse	ruptured membranes Signal of onset of labor
agakomere ko mugisusu	anal fistula An opening in the skin that tracts to the anal canal thus causing some fecal material to leak from the opening in the skin.
agakomokomo	brain stem An organ that consists of the medulla oblongata, pons and midbrain. (base of the brain)
agakomokomo	occiput Back of the head.

115

Kirundi	English
agakomokomo	cerebellum The part of the brain in the posterior portion of the skull that controls muscle coordination and movement.
agapfukahaha	pleura The serous membrane lining each lung.
agasaho gahingura amazi yumwana	amnion The membrane lining the placenta which produces the amniotic fluid.
agasaho ko mumutima	atrium Referring to a chamber used as an entrance, as in the entrance to the heart.
agasaho k'umusenyi k'urusogi	appendix An appendage of the cecum.
agasama	chicken pox, varicella A viral disease characterized by extremely pruritus blisters over the entire body.
agasama	measles A childhood viral, infectious disease exhibited by rash and fever.
agasama	varicella A virus that causes chickenpox and shingles. Also called herpes zoster.
agasendabageni	cheekbone
agasendabageni	maxilla The upper jaw that also forms the inferior portion of the orbit and part of the nose.
agashangara (c'ikivukano)	congenital syphilis Passed to the child in utero, the child may have failure to thrive, fever and a flattened bridge of the nose.
agashangara; isofisi	syphilis A infectious disease caused by Treponema pallidum that causes a painless penile ulcer in the primary stage but can lead to irreversible brain damage in the untreated tertiary stage.
agashinge	lancet A small sharp instrument used to obtain a drop of blood for testing.
agashitsi	chills Sensation of coldness.
agasimba	bug Insect.
agasaho kimbuto zumugore	ovary One of a paired of female reproductive glands containing oocytes.
agaswende; mburugu	gonorrhea A sexually transmitted disease that is exhibited by purulent discharge from the vagina or penis.
agaswime	feminine pad Gauze specially designed to absorb menstrual flow.
agaswime	sanitary napkin Cloth or synthetic material used to absorb menstrual blood.
agatabu kicandarwa	vaccine certificate A document that denotes what vaccines have been received by the holder.
agatambara ko guhanagura amaraso bariko barabaga	sponge Sterile fabric used to soak up fluid during surgery.
agateka	right Justice or fairness.(noun)
agatosi	blemish A small mark on one's skin.
agatwe	apex The highest point of something.
aka	free from Lacking or absent.
akababaro	shock Surprise or astonishment. (startled)
akabonge	depression A medical condition exhibited by profound despondency.
akabonge	sadness The state of being sad.

Kirundi	English
akabonge	trauma A physical injury or emotional shock.
akabuye kaba mu mugende w'indurwe	gallstone Calculus produced in the bile duct or gallbladder.
akabuye ko mu ndugu	calculus A stone of minerals that can lead to the blockage of the bile duct or ureters.
akagufa kinyongera	exostosis A bony prominence growing from the surface of a bone.
akahanzi	headache Cephalgia.
akakangavya	epididymitis Inflammation of the duct that moves sperm from the testis to the vas deferens. (unilateral testicular swelling)
akamakama	drop by drop Expression meaning little by little.
akameme	epigastrium The section of the abdomen that overlies the stomach.
akamirampeke	Adam's apple A prominence on the anterior neck caused by the thyroid cartilage of the larynx.
akanogo	cavity Pouch or chamber.
akanovera	after-taste The sensation of a prolonged savor following eating/drinking.
akanwa	mouth The orifice on the lower part of the face.
akanyuzi ko kugenyera	umbilical tape Material used to tie off the umbilical cord prior to cutting it after the baby is born.
akaranda; ibihara	smallpox Variola.
akaranga k ubuntu	personality Qualities that form a person's unique character.
akarimirimi	epiglottis Tissue at the base of the tongue that covers the trachea when one swallows.
akaringoti ko mugutwi	eustachian tube The muscular canal that connects the tympanic membrane with the pharynx
akasambangwiga	angioedema Also called angioneurotic edema, it is caused by a histamine reaction. It can produce welts in mild cases but in severe cases can cause swelling of the lips and tongue.
akasate	hemiplegia Paralysis of one side of the body.
akasokoro	hematuria The presence of blood in the urine.
akayiko gato	tablespoon An eating utensil that holds 15milliliters of fluid.
akaziba kinda	xiphoid process The inferior segment of the sternum.
akazu ka sugumwe	toilet Device used during urination/defecation.
akazuyazi	tepid Lukewarm.
akigoro	effort Attempt or endeavor.
akuma gafasha kumva	hearing aid A device that fits in the ear used to amplify sound.
akuma ko gupima umurindi wamaraso	sphygmomanometer Device for measuring blood pressure.
akuma ko gusiga umuti kurukoba	applicator A device used to apply a topical medication.
akuma ko kuringaniza uruvyaro ko mu gitereko	intrauterine contraceptive device (IUD) A device used to physically prevent the implantation of a fertilized ovum.
amabekire	crutches Long metal or wooden sticks used for support while walking.

117

Kirundi	English
amaberebere	breast milk
amacinya	dysentery A severe form of diarrhea with blood and mucous in the stool.
amacyinya	hematochezia Presence of blood in the excrement.
amada	lice Plural for louse, a small parasite that lives on the skin. Pediculus humanus capitis is a head louse.
amafata y'ukwisiga	balm A topical medical preparation.
amafata y'ukwisiga	ointment A petroleum jelly based topical medication.
amafinya	lumbar Referring to the spinal region inferior to the thoracic spine.
amagage	tonsils A rounded mass of lymphoid tissue, most commonly referring to the pharyngeal tonsil.
amagage	uvula A fleshy pendent at the back of the soft palate.
amaganya	anxiety Nervousness or unease.
amagara	health The state of being free of illness.
amagara y'inyo	anal sphincter Ring of striated muscle fibers surrounding the anus.
amagara y'umukenyezi imbere yuko asama	pre-conception health The health habits, medications and nutritional status of a woman before becoming pregnant.t
amagizo	gait The way one walks.
amagufa	skeleton Internal bony framework.
amagume	crisis A turning point in the treatment of a disease.
amaguru y'imbango	bow-legged Synonym for genu varum.
amaguru y'inkika	genu varum A condition exhibited by the knees turning outward, commonly referred to as bowleg.
amahasa biteye kumwe	identical twins Twins from the same zygote.
amahere	exanthema A rash that accompanies a disease or fever.
amahere	rash Exanthema or urticaria.
amahere	skin rash Dermal exanthema.
amahere y'inyonko	cold sore A perioral blister caused by herpes simplex.
amakenga	apprehensive A fear that something unpleasant will happen.
amama akoroka kumunota	drops per minute Refers to iv fluid rate.
amangati	eructation Belch or burp.
amanyezi	stomach contents, undigested
amapfungo	fasting Absence of caloric intake for a specified period.
amara	duodenum The portion of the small bowel between the stomach and jejunum.
amara	intestines A general term used for the section of bowel from the stomach to the anus.
amarakaraka	glottis Essentially the vocal structure, including the true vocal cords and the opening between them.
amaraso	blood Plasma containing erythrocytes, leukocytes and platelets.
amaraso ava ku'mutima, yamare ashike h'inyuma y'umuwiri	abdominal girth Waist circumference.
amarira	tear As in a vaginal tear after childbirth.

Kirundi	English
amarwi	incisor Sharp-edged tooth; humans have four incisors.
amasambambwika	mumps A contagious viral disease that is exhibited by parotid swelling and puts males at risk for sterility. Also called epidemic parotitis.
amashanya	jaw Mandible.
amashanya	mandible The lower jaw.
amashesheti	socks Worn on the feet before one puts on shoes.
amashira	pus Thick yellow or green opaque liquid as seen with infection.
amashoka	noon The 12 o'clock mid-day hour.
amashure	education Instruction or guidance.
amasinizite	sinusitis Inflammation of the sinuses.
amaso arirashye	hemeralopia Night blindness.
amaso arirashye	night blindness Common term for nyctalopia, it refers to low vision with reduced illumination, often seen with Vitamin A deficiency.
amaso atukura	icterus Yellowing of the skin and sclerae because of excess bilirubin.
amaso;uruhanga	face Anterior aspect of the head from the forehead to the chin.
amasonzi	nipples The small projections on the breast thru which milk is secreted in females.
amasozi	lacrimal fluid Fluid secreted by the lacrimal gland.
amasozi	tears Fluid expelled from the eyes during crying.
amata	cow's milk
amatako (itako)	buttocks (buttock) The bilateral region covering the gluteal muscles.
amate	saliva The watery liquid secreted by the salivary glands.
amate	spit A term used to describe saliva that is ejected from the mouth.
amavuta	fat A greasy or oiling substance naturally occurring in the body.
amavuta yo mu mubiri	cholesterol A compound or its derivatives are found in cell membranes and precursors to hormones but high levels can cause atherosclerosis.
amavuta yo mumavi	synovial fluid The fluid that surrounds, for example, the knee within a capsule.
amavyi; umwanda mukuru; uho kwituma	stool Feces, excrement.
amazi	drinking water Water clean enough to ingest orally.
amazi	water A colorless, odorless liquid.
amazi asa n amata yo mumubiri,ahingura abasirikare bumubiri	lymph A transparent and sometimes opalescent fluid that flows in the lymph channels.
amazi ava mumubiri	secretion The discharge of substances from cells or glands.
amazi yo mubihimba vyirondoka	smegma A thick curdled secretion found around the clitoris and the prepuce.
amazi yo muruti rw umugongo	cerebrospinal fluid (CSF) The fluid between the pia mater and arachnoid membrane.

Kirundi	English
Amazi yo muruti rwumugongo	CSF Abbreviation for cerebrospinal fluid.
amazi yumwana aseseka umwanya muremure	prolonged rupture of the membranes Rupture of the membranes more than 24 hours before delivery.
ambura; vanamo impuzu	undress Take one's clothes off; disrobe.
amenyo y'amaterano	dentures A frame that holds artificial teeth.
Amosozi	eye drops Liquid applied to eyes for various medical problems.
amuti wubushuhe	antipyretic Medication used to treat fever.
ankirositome	hookworm A parasitic infection of the family Strongylidae that can cause anemia.
aramugaye; ubumuga	paralysis Inability to move one or more extremities.
arawaye mu muhogo	tonsillitis Inflammation of the tonsils.
areze amaboko	passive Not achieved through active effort.
ari mu gupfa	moribund Near death.
arwaye mu mutwe	insane A term not used in formal medical evaluations that when used by a layperson means a serious mental illness.
asima	asthma An inflammatory disease of the lungs noteworthy because of reversible airway obstruction.
ata inabi (indwara itagira uwubi)	benign Not harmful. (benign condition)
ata nkeka	indeed As a matter of fact.
atakimenyetso cindwara	asymptomatic The absence of symptoms.
atazi gusoma n'ukwandika	illiterate Unable to read or write.
bawasiri	hemorrhoids Engorgement of the veins in the anus or rectum.
bibera icarimwe	simultaneous Occurring at the same time.
bidakenewe	trivial Of little importance or value.
bidasumbanye	equilibrium When opposing forces are in balance.
bidatumberanye	asymmetry Lack of symmetry.
bifise umukondo umwe	concentric Referring to circles or arcs that share the same center.
bijanye	compatible To coexist without problems.
bijanye na.	related to Causally connected.
bike kurusha	less A smaller amount.
bikenewe	underlying Causative, unexposed, or fundamental.
Birariziose	Bilharzia Historical name of a genus of flukes or nematodes now known as Schistosoma.
birariziyoze	schistosomiasis A condition, sometimes known as bilharzia, which involves infestation with flukes of the genus Schistosoma.
birenduka	sludge A viscous fluid.
bitarimwo	fair Equitable.
bitumbiri	genital ambiguity A disorder of sexual development in which the genitalia are not sufficiently developed to tell clearly if the person is male or female.
buhoro	slight Minor or small.
buhoro	slow Unhurried.

Kirundi	English
buri misi ibiri	every other day On alternate days.
burimwaka	yearly Occurring once each year.
ca buri ndwi	weekly That which occurs every seven days.
cacerewe	late A time later than expected.
cagutse	widespread Encompassing or spanning.
catayigihe	obsolete No longer in use; antiquated.
chaleur	hot Very warm.
cica	lethal Deadly.
cihuta	abrupt Suddenly or hastily.
co hagati	medial Situated toward the midline.
co hanyuma	posterior Further back in position; opposite of anterior.
co mu bwenge	mental Cognitive or psychological.
co mu mbavu	lateral Referring to the side of the body.
co mu nyama	intramuscular Within a muscle.
corosha	lubricant Emollient.
coroshe	mild Slight, nominal.
cumye	dry Absence of moisture.
c'akaronda	hereditary That which is transmitted genetically
c'amagara meza	healthy In good health.
c'icubirizi	unexpected Unforeseen.
c'ighimbano	artificial Not natural produced.
c'imbere mu gitereko	intrauterine Within the uterus.
c'imbere w'umutwe	intracranial Within the cranial vault.
c'imbere yo kwibaruka	prenatal Referring to the time prior to birth.
c'imbere y'inda	intraabdominal Within the abdominal cavity.
c'imbere y'ubutinyanka	premenstrual Occurring prior to the onset of menstruation.
c'imisi yose	every day Each day.
c'impera	last Final.
c'inyuma y'ibagwa	post-operative Referring to the time after an operation.
c'itegeko	mandatory Obligatory.
c'ubuntu	human Homo sapien.
c'ubwoya	hirsutism Abnormal growth on hair on a person's face and body.
c'ukuri	right Correct, accurate (adjective)
diphtheria (ikirato)	diphtheria A contagious bacterial disease characterized by a grey membrane on the pharynx along with respiratory or cutaneous symptoms; caused by Corynebacterium diphtheriae.
dukeya twa inkari	dribble, to To slowly, drip-by-drip, release urine for example.
gahembe	bubonic plague A form of plague exhibited by the formation of buboes.
genda ku bitaro	go to the hospital, to
genda kwa muganga	go to the doctor, to

121

Kirundi	English
genda kwa muganga kaurikirane ivyerekeye amagara yawe n'amagara y'ibondo utwaye	prenatal care The medical care received after becoming pregnant and before childbirth.
gica mu mutsi w'amaraso	intravenous Within a vein.
gifushe	blunt Having a flat or rounded end.
gihushanye	contradictory Two elements that are inconsistent.
gihuye na	consistent Compatible with something or congruous with.
gihwahutse	light Not heavy.
gihwekereye	quiescent A time of inactivity.
gikabije	drastic Having significant effect.
gikaze	severe Intense or very great.
gikonje	frozen Past participle of to freeze. Freeze: turn a liquid into a solid.
gikora neza	efficacious Effective.
gikurikira	next The following or upcoming.
gikuru	essential Crucial or necessary.
gikwiriye	convenient Opportune or well-timed.
gikwiye	adequate Sufficient.
gishikana ku rupfu	fatal Lethal.
gishobora kwirindwa	avoidable That which can be stopped or inhibited.
gishusha	analogous To resemble or be similar to.
gisigura gukiza indwara	heal, to To treat or to cure.
gitaburuye	gaping Wide open.
gitezura	emollient Having softening or soothing qualities.
gitose	wet Covered in moisture.
guca umutwe	decapitate, to The physical separation of the head from the body.
guceka	shake, to To tremble uncontrollably.
gucikana	expire, to To die.
gucira	expectorate,to To expulsion of sputum associated with a cough.
gucira amate	spit,to To expectorate or expel saliva from the mouth.
gufata	cancel, to To stop or revoke.
gufata umuti	take medication, to
gufatana	coagulate, to The formation of a clot.
gufatwa n'umutima	heart attack Common term for myocardial infarction.
gufatwa n'umutima	myocardial infarction The death of myocardial tissue as a result of an interruption in flow to the region supplied by a coronary vessel.
gufudika	blurt out, to To speak without considering the repercussions.
gufuhagira	snore, to To snore or grunt while breathing during sleep. (a snore)
gufunga	close, to
gufyfoza	whistle, to To make a high pitch noise by forcing air through the lips.
guhagarara	stand, to To stop or to be upright

Kirundi	English
guhagarika guhema	respiratory arrest Cessation of breathing.
guhakana	deny, to To reject or repudiate.
guhamangira	bearing down As in during labor.
guhanura	advise, to To give counsel.
guharira	argue, to To debate or reason. (quarrel)
guharura	count, to To determine a number.
guharura umubiri	bruise, to Common term for to cause ecchymosis.
guhekenya	masticate,to To chew.
guhema cane	hyperventilation Rapid and deep respirations.
guhema itama rimwe	sniff,to Short, rapid nasal inhalation. (or to smell)
guhema nabi	orthopnea The inability to breath comfortably except in the upright position.
guhema nabi	stridor An abnormal, high-pitched, musical sound caused by an obstruction in the larynx or stenosis of the vocal cords.
guhema; guhumeka	breathe, to The act of respiration.
guhemuka	expire,to To exhale.
guhengama	biased Prejudiced.
guhenuka	collapse To have a physical or mental breakdown.
guheraheza	accomplish, to Achieve.
guheza	achieve, to To complete something one was striving for.
guhezagirika	hyperpnea Abnormal increase in rate and depth of respiration.
guhezagirika	tachypnea Breathing faster than normal.
guhezera	wheeze,to
guhimbura	brace, to Application of a splint.
guhindukiriza inyuma	pronation Turning posteriorly. When the hand is pronated, it is turned medially until the palm is facing posteriorly (when the body was initially in the anatomic position).
guhindukiza amaso cane	Rapid Eye Movement The movement of a person's eyes during this period of sleep.
guhindukiza amaso cane mwitiro	REM (rapid eye movement) sleep This period of sleep is associated with irregular respirations and heart rate, involuntary movements and dreaming.
guhindura	adjust, to To modify a plan.
guhindura ipansoma	dressing, to change a To place a new dressing on a wound.
guhingura isabuni	saponify,to The creation of soap from oil using an alkali.
guhinyuza	check for, to
guhitwa	diarrhea, to have (verb) The act of having diarrhea.
guhonoka	bear, to To give birth to a child.
guhora	silent,to be Absence of noise or no indication of something.
guhotora	torsion Refers to twisting. Testicular torsion is the twisting of the spermatic cord that can lead to ischemia and gangrene of the testicle.
guhuma	blind, to be To have an absence of visual perception.

123

Kirundi	English
guhumaguza	blink, to To open and close the eyelid rapidly.
guhunyereza	squint, to To look at something with the eyes partially closed.
guhurira	itch, to To have a sensation of pruritis.
guhushagirika	stagger, to To walk in an unsteady fashion.
guhuza ibitsina	sexual intercourse The act of copulation.
guhuza imiryango	marital counseling Therapy aimed at marriage reconciliation.
gukama	decrease Becoming smaller or fewer.
gukama amaraso	iron-deficiency anemia A microcytic anemia.
gukama amate	aptyalism Diminished or absence of saliva.
gukama intanga	aspermia Absence of sperm.
gukama isukari mumubiri	hypoglycemia Abnormally low blood sugar.
gukamya	desiccation The act of drying up.
gukanya	hypothermia Lower than normal temperature.
gukanya	squeeze, to To apply pressure.
gukashuka	strain,to As in a muscle strain.
gukata ikirimi	uvulectomy Excision of the uvula.
gukatika impemu	apnea Absence of respiration.
gukeha impemu mumubiri	anoxia Reduced oxygen levels in body tissues.
gukenera birengeye urugero	crave,to An unusually strong urge for something.
gukenerwa gu...	owing to On account of.
gukerebuka	wise,to be Possessing much knowledge.
gukikira	around, to be To be on every side of.
gukira	recover from a grave illness, to
gukira bukebuke	remission A decrease in severity or a temporary resolution.
gukiriza	lift, to Raise to a higher level.
gukomera	strong,to be Having the power to move heavy objects.
gukomereka	injure, to be To hurt or to wound.
gukona	castrate, to Excision of the gonads.
gukongatara kwamaso	odontalgia Tooth pain.
gukonya	flex To bend.
Gukora ingoma y ugutwi	tympanoplasty Restoration of the tympanic membrane's continuity.
gukorako	affect The expression of emotions or feelings.
gukorako	touch,to Tactile stimulation.
gukorakora	palpate,to The assessment of the body with the use of one's hands.
gukoresha ukuryo cane	right-handed Having a preference to use the right hand.
Gukoropa mu bihimba vyirondoka	curettage Removal of tissues from a cavity.
gukorora	cough, to
Gukorora amaraso	hemoptysis Expectoration of blood.
Gukorora imbanyi,	abortion, inevitable Presence of cervical dilation or ruptured membranes in a pregnancy where the baby is not viable.

Kirundi	English
gukorora imbere yo kuvuga utomora	clear one's throat, to To cough lightly in attempt to speak more clearly.
gukoroza imbanyi	induced abortion Surgical or medical evacuation of the fetus.
gukosora amagufa yatiriganye	reduction Return of a dislocated joint or fractured bone to its proper position.
gukosora umuringoti nsozantaga	urethroplasty Surgical repair of the urethra.
gukoyora	voiding The act of urinating.
gukubita kurugero rwo hejuru kandi rujanye	throb, to The beat with strong regular rhythm.
gukura	remove,to The act of removing something.
gukuraho	clearance The process of removing something.
gukurako ikintu	debridement Trimming the dead tissue adjacent to a wound.
gukurugutura	cerumen impaction, to clean out Cleansing of external ear canal because it is full of wax resulting in hearing loss.
gukwegura	extend, to To expand or stretch out.
gukweka	pull, to To exert force on something.
gupasuka	rupture An instance of bursting suddenly.
gupfa	dead, to be Deceased. (dead person)
gupfa	die, to To stop living, to expire.
gupfukama	kneel,to Being on one's knees as in the prayer position.
gupfukamisha amavi n inkokora	knee elbow position Knees and elbows are on the table and the chest is in the air.
gupfuna	nose, blow the
gupima	screening An evaluation as part of a methodical study.
gupima	weigh, to
gupima intanga	semen analysis Evaluation of semen used as part of a fertility workup.
gupima inyubakwa itunganirizwamwo ibipimo	laboratory test
gupima inzoga mumpwemu	breath test (for alcohol) A check of alcohol level by testing exhaled air.
gupima mugisusu nurutoki	rectal digital examination Use of a gloved finger to assess the rectal vault.
gupima ubwonko n'imitsi (gupima icumvirizo)	neurology test
gupima umukoyo	urinalysis Chemical and microscopic examination of the urine.
gupima umutima	echocardiogram Use of ultrasound to evaluate the heart.
gupimisha imbanyi	pregnancy test, to get a
gusa, or kungana	symmetry Being equally bilaterally.
gusama inda	conception The act of an egg being fertilized by sperm.
gusama inda; kuremerwa	pregnant, to be
gusamaza	expect, to To suppose or presume.
gusamba	agony, to be in Anguish or torment.
gusamba	spasm,to have a An involuntary contraction of muscles.

125

Kirundi	English
gusanga amaraso mugasaho gapfuka umutima	hemopericardium Abnormal presence of blood in the pericardium.
gusanza	scatter The degree to which repeated measurements differ.
gusasatwa munda	rebound A term used to describe a type of tenderness found with peritonitis.
gusatura mu nda mu kukuvyaza	cesarean section Incision of the abdominal and uterine walls in order to deliver a fetus when natural delivery is not possible.
gusaza	older Being around more than compared with another.
gusaza kwamagufa	osteoporosis Loss of bone substance because the osteoblasts fail to produce bone matrix.
guseruka	deterioration Worsening in one's medical condition.
gushanyuka	apart, to be Separated by a distance.
gushinyaguriza	abuse, to (verbal abuse)
gushira mu ngiro	implementation The process of putting a plan into effect.
gushoboza	qualify To become eligible by fulfilling a necessary standard.
gushona	running suture A method of sewing a wound in which there is a knot at each end and continuous otherwise.
gushona umubiri	anastomosis Surgical formation of a connection between two previously separate parts.
gusiba	abstain, to To give up or to stop.
gusiba y'intoboro	imperforate Lack of an opening. An infant with an imperforate anus has a congenital defect with no anal opening.
gusimbagurika umutima	tachycardia Heart rate higher than physiologic normal.
gusinzira	sleep,to The act of sleeping
gusinziriza	hypnotic Sleep inducing agent.
gusinziriza	sedative A medication used to facilitate sleep or calm a person.
gusoba	urinate,to
gusoba amashira	pyuria Presence of purulent material in the urine.
Gusoba duke	oliguria Abnormally low urine output.
gusoba n'ijoro	nocturia Urination at night.
gusohoka	eversion To turn outward.
gusohoka	leakage Unintentional escape of gas or fluid.
gusohoka ibitaro	hospital discharge To leave the hospital.
gusohora amashira	pyorrhea Emission of pus.
gusohora umwuka	evacuation The emptying of an organ of fluids or gas.
gusokora	raise, to To lift or bring up.
gusoma dukeya	sip, to To slowly take small drinks of a fluid.
gusoma nturi	drown,to The process of dying from submerging in and inhaling water.
gusomora	dress,to To apply gauze to a wound.
gusubira inyuma	retrograde Referring to backward movement.
gusubiramwo	regurgitation 1. Backflow of blood in the heart. 2. Movement of gastric contents into the mouth.

Kirundi	English
gusurira	flatus,to pass To expel air from the anus.
gusurira	pass, flatus to To release bowel gas from the anus.
gusuzuma	auscultate, to The act of listening to sounds emanating from the body.
gusuzuma ko	ensure, to To make certain of.
gusuzumisha amabere imishwarara (x)	mammogram X ray imaging of the breasts to look for breast cancer.
gusuzumisha urwinjiriro rw'igitereko	pap smear Microscopic exam of cells from a swab of the cervix.
guta igihe	outdated Something that has passed the expiration date.
guta ubwenge	unconsciousness Unable to respond to sensory stimuli.
gutabuka imitsi yo mw iteranirizo ry itako	groin pull A muscle strain in the inguinal region.
gutahura	comprehend, to To understand.
gutahura	lengthen,to To make or become longer.
gutakana	yell, to To speak in a loud tone.
gutakaze	decline As in a decrease in status or health.
gutamira	mouthful To take a large quantity of something in one's mouth.
gutamya	worry, to To fret or have unease.
gutandukana mu ngingo	dislocation The displacement of a bone when referring to an articulation. (sprain, dislocate, startle)
gutapfuna	chew, to Masticate.
gutata	conflict Dispute or disagreement.
gutera amaraso	transfusion Administration of blood products intravenously.
gutera igihimba c'umubiri	transplant,to To move a body part from one location to another.
gutera indihaguzi	beat As in heart beat.
gutera umugere	kick, to To strike an object with one's foot.
gutera urushinge	infuse,to The injection of fluid into tissue or a vein.
gutera urushinge	inject,to The act of a needle being inserted into a body. (given injection)
guterura	rape,to Forced sexual relations.
gutetemera	ague A term used to describe recurrent fever and shivering typically associated with malaria.
gutetemera	tremble from fever, to
gutetemera	tremor Involuntary contraction and relaxation of small muscle groups.
gutezura	relieve, to (pain) To make less severe.
gutimba kwumupfu	rigor mortis The normal stiffening of the muscles and joints that occurs a few hours after death.
gutimba umubiri wose	quadriplegia Paralysis of all four extremities.
Gutimbsha	anesthesia Loss of sensation.
gutinya amazi	hydrophobia Abnormal fear of water.
gutinya umuco	photophobia Abnormal sensitivity to light.
gutinya; kwikanga	fear, to have Fright or trepidation.

Kirundi	English
gutobeka	contaminate, to To make impure by exposing to an polluted agent.
gutora	choose, to To make an election or decision.
gutubwenge	prostration Profound exhaustion.
gutukura	blush, to To have an increased volume of blood flow to one's face causing a red tint to the skin.
gutura amangati	belch, to Eructation.
guturika	skin disease that causes red spots,to have
Guturumbura amaso	exophthalmos Protrusion of one or both eyeballs.
gutwenga	laugh, to
hafi	near In close proximity.
hafi y amazuru	paranasal Situated adjacent to the nose.
hafi y iteranirizo ry amagufa	juxta-articular Positioned near a joint.
hafi yigisusu	pararectal Adjacent to the rectum.
hagati	center A point equidistant from all sides.
hagati y amagufa yomugikiriza	intercostal Area between the ribs
hahandi nyene	ipsilateral On the same side.

Kirundi	English
hamwe	equal The same or uniform.
hasi	inferior The lower aspect.
hedzjuru ry'ikirenge	instep The medial aspect of the foot between the ankle and the ball of the foot.
hejuru	above
hejuru	superior In a position above something else.
hejuru	proximal Situated closer to the center of the body (opposed to that which is farther away, as in distal).
hejuru yibipimo fatiro	greater than normal Above normal.
hepfo	below Under.
hepfo	down In a lower position.
hose	every Each or all possible.
hugaye	obstructed To be blocked or halted.
ibavu	blister Common term for bulla.
ibavu	callosity Callus; thickened hardened skin.
ibere	breast Mammary tissue including the areola.
ibgena	canine teeth Located between the incisors and premolars.
ibice nkingiramubiri biri mu bigeze amaraso	leukocyte A white blood cell.
ibicurane; ibiseru	rhinorrhea Abundant nasal mucosal drainage.
ibifaranga	tinea barbae Ringworm on the face in the region a man shaves.
ibigatu	tinea pedis Ringworm of the feet, a fungal infection.
ibigero	puberty The time when adolescents become capable of sexual reproduction.
ibihagati	emotion An intense feeling.
ibihanga	toothless person
ibihara	German measles (rubella) A contagious viral infection.
ibihara	rubella Also called German measles, it is characterized by a rash, fever, headache.
Ibihatane	impaction, tooth A tooth that does not erupt because adjacent teeth prevent it.
ibihimba vy'irondoka	genitalia Genitals.
ibikoresho	equipment Apparatus or instrument.
ibikorwa vy'ubtabazi	first aid The initial treatment after an injury.
ibimirimiro	angina pectoris Exercise induced myocardial ischemia.
ibinini vyo kumira	contraceptives, oral A medication taken by mouth by a woman to prevent pregnancy.
ibintoro	framboesia; yaws An endemic tropical disease caused by Treponema pertenue.
ibinyanya	paresthesia An abnormal sensation usually described as pins and needles.

Kirundi	English
ibinyoro	yaws A tropical disease characterized by ulcers on the extremities, caused by Treponema pertenue.
Ibirashi	eye discharge Conjunctival discharge.
Ibirashi	discharge, postpartum vaginal The secretions noted after delivery.
ibirimwo	content What something is made up of.
ibiro vy umubiri	body weight Relative mass as measured in kilograms or pounds.
ibisahuzi	seizure An episode of tonic/clonic movement noted in epilepsy.
ibisazi	rage Uncontrollable anger.
ibise	labor pains The intermittent pain associated with uterine contractions.
ibisebe biterwa n'isuna	canker sore An ulceration, usually of the mouth or lips.
ibisereka	tinea corporis Ringworm of the body, a fungal infection.
ibisereka	tinea cruris Ringworm in the inguinal region, a fungal infection.
ibitaro	hospital Acute care medical/surgical facility.
ibumoso;ibubamfu	left
ibungwe ry'iryinyo	dental caries Decay of teeth.
ibutumbi	swelling An abnormal enlarged from fluid collection.
ibyobezabwenge	drug A medication, sometimes with negative connotation.
Icaguzo	dilator An instrument that dilates.
icandaga	inoculation Injection with a vaccine to provide immunity.
icigwa c'ibinyabuzima	biology The study of living organisms.
icigwa c'indwara z'ikiza	epidemiology The study of the incidence, development and control of disease.
icirori	mirror A device used for reflecting an image.
icirwa cibikoko	zoology The study of animals.
icizigiro	confidence Self-assurance.
icombo abagwaye bitumamwo	bedpan A metal or plastic vestibule one sits on while in bed to defecate.
icuma	iron An element found in hemoglobin.
Icuma bakoresha mu gukoropa mumubiri	curette The instrument used during a curettage.
icuma co gufata	tongs A medical device used for holding or grasping.
icuma co gukosora indwara y umusipa	truss A synthetic device for containing a hernia within the abdomen.
Icuma co kubaga	forceps A surgical instrument, commonly called tweezers.
icuma gihingura umuti wo mumahaha	nebulizer A device used for transforming a liquid into a fine mist for inhalation as in nebulized albuterol for an acute exacerbation of asthma.
icuma gipima itera ry'umutima	stethoscope Instrument used to listen to the heart and lungs.
icuma gitandukanya inyama mukubaga	retractor A device for pulling back tissue during surgery.
icuma gitanga umwuka	respirator A device used to artificially ventilate a patient.
icuma kibundikira abana	incubator A warming device for infants.

Kirundi	English
icumba	ventricle 1. One of two chambers of the heart. 2. The four inter-connected cavities in the center of the brain.
icumba c abarwayi	ward A section of a hospital where patients reside.
icumba vyahariwe abarwaye indwara zandukira	isolation ward A ward where patients with infectious disease are housed.
icumbi	accommodation A term used to describe the ability of the eye to adjust to various distances.
icunyunyu ca Plomb	lead An element with an atomic number of 82.
icupa	bottle A container used for the storage of liquids.
icuya	perspiration The process of sweating.
icuya	sweat Moisture exuded through the pores of the skin.
icyago; icaduka; igisida	accident
icyungisho	splint A rigid support used to immobilize and extremity.
idururu	vulva The external genitalia of the female.
idzjicyo riramenese	cornea prolapse Protrusion of the cornea from injury.
idzjicyo ry'ikirenge	talus The most superior tarsal bone that articulates with the tibia.
ifagitire	bill A financial statement that indicates how much one owes.
ifigo	kidney One of two glandular organs that form urine.
iforomasiyo	pharmacy A business that sells prescription medication.
ifundo	muscle, calf
ifungura	dilution The process of making a weaker solution.
ifuro	foam A mass of small bubbles in a liquid.
ifuro	froth Covered with a mass of small bubbles.
ifuti	error Mistake or inaccuracy.
ifyondekara ry imitsi yuruti rwumugongo	cord compression Pressure being applied to the spinal cord.
igabanganya	cleavage A sharp division or demarcation.
igabanuka	shortening Notable for having a shorter length.
igabanywa mudusaho twinshi	loculated Divided into small cavities.
iganya	anguish Significant mental or physical pain.
igaruka	dilatation The process of becoming wider or larger.
igarukagaruka	frequency Rate of occurrence.
igice	half Divided in two.
igice c ijisho	conjunctiva The membrane that lines the eyelid.
igice c umwanya	half-life The time a drug decreases its effect in half over time.
Igice cubwonko	dura mater The outermost covering of the brain and spinal cord.
igice c'ububoko gifatanye n'urutugu	forearm Segment of the arm from the elbow to wrist.
igice kibonerana co mujisho	cornea The transparent segment located at the anterior part of the eye.
igiciro	cost The fee or penalty.
igifasha umurwayi kugenda	walker A metal frame used to facilitate walking.
igifuka	pleurisy Inflammation of the pleura.

131

Kirundi	English
igihe c amasaha 24	circadian Referring to a 24 hour period.
igihe cinyuma yibisahuzi	postictal The period of time after a seizure.
igihe ntarengwa	deadline Cutoff date.
igihemesho co kwa muganga	non-rebreather mask A type of oxygen mask used to deliver a higher oxygen concentration.
igihere	bedbug Cimex lectularius. A small insect that is parasitic and hides in clothing or bedding.
igihima curuti rwumugongo	epidural The space around the dura of the spinal cord.
igihimba c ubwonko	pia mater The first layer of three covering the brain and spinal cord.
igihimba cijisho	aqueous humor The fluid between the cornea and lens, anterior to the globe.
igihimba co mugitereko	endometrium The mucous membrane lining of the uterus.
igihimba co mugutwi	cochlea The essential organ of hearing which is in a spiral form.
igihimba co muzuru	septum A wall separating two chambers, the nasal septum for example.
igihimba cubwonko	hypothalamus Located inferior to the thalamus it controls visceral activities, water balance, temperature and sleep.
igihimba cubwonko	subarachnoid The layer of the brain covering between the arachnoid and pia mater.
igihimba cumutima	myocardium The middle layer of the heart wall.
igihimba gihingura amosozi	lacrimal Referring to the secretion of tears.
igihimba gisigaye	stump Term used to designate what remains of an amputated extremity.
igihimba nterano cokwivi	prosthesis An artificial body part. (above the knee) [below the knee]
igihimba ntunganyambuto	gonad A testis or an ovary.
igihogo	brown Coffee-colored.
igihogohogo	endotracheal Within the trachea.
igihogohogo	trachea The ringed canal between the pharynx and bronchi.
igihogohogo; umuhogo	esophagus The muscular tube that connects the throat to the stomach.
igihume	anencephaly The congenital absence of the cranial vault and cerebral hemispheres.
igihume	acephalous A absence of a head.
igihute	boil Small abscess or furuncle.
igihute	abscess A localized collection of pus.
Igihute co mugitigu	liver abscess A localized collection of pus in the liver.
igihute co mumagage	quinsy Peritonsillar inflammation or abscess.
igihute co mumahaha	empyema A collection of purulent material in a body cavity, usually referring to a thoracic empyema.
igihute co mumugongo	spinal cord abscess A localized collection of purulent material in or adjacent to the spinal cord.
igihute co munda	intraabdominal abscess A collection of pus in the abdomen.
igihute co murwara	paronychia Inflammation of the tissue bordering a fingernail
igihuteco mukannwa	peritonsillar abscess
igikakwe	perspiration from armpit (or bad body odor)

Kirundi	English
igikangaga	tapeworm A parasitic, intestinal flatworm.
igikanu	neck, back of (nape) Posterior aspect of the neck.
igikere	frog A tailless amphibian that is short with long hind legs for jumping.
igikiriza	chest Thorax.
igikiriza	thorax The part of the body between the neck and abdomen.
igikomere	sore An ulcer or lesion.
igikomere c umuzingi	wheal A circumscribed urticarial lesion.
igikomere co kuremerwa	pressure ulcer Loss in skin integrity due to a portion of the body being in the same position for too long and possibly other factors.
igikomere cuwarashwe	gunshot wound An penetrating injury sustained from a bullet.
igikomere kiregeye	stab wound An injury occurring with a sharp object.
igikonjo	hand The upper extremity distal to the wrist.
igikonjo	hand, dorsum Back of hand.
igikonjo	wrist The articulation of the hand and radius/ulna.
igikonjo ciburyo	hand, right
igikonyo	apathy Lack of interest in one's environment or indifference.
igikororwa	phlegm Sputum.
igikororwa	sputum A mixture of respiratory tract secretions and saliva.
igikumu	agreement Accordance in opinion or feeling.
igikuri	dwarf Abnormally small person.
igipfamatwi	deaf Absence of the sense of hearing. (deaf person)
igipfungu	hazy Cloudy.
igipimabushuhe	thermometer A device used to measure temperature.
Igipimo c urugero rwubwenge bwindembe	Glasgow coma scale A scale used to grade one's level of consciousness with a score of 3 being totally unresponsive and a score of 15 being normal.
igipimo cibiro nukwo umuntu angana	body surface area Dubois formula is: (weight in kilograms)to the 0.425th power x (height in centimeters) to the 0.725th power x 0.007184.
igipimo co hejuru cumurindi wamaraso	systolic Referring to systole or that which occurs during systole.
igipimo co kuraba ko umurwayi wimitsi ashobora gutembereza agatsinstiri kuva kwivi gushika kukirenge iburyo n ibubamfu.	heel-shin test (heel to knee to toe test) A test of position sense and coordination; one moves the heel of one foot from the knee on the other foot down to the foot.
igipimo co kwa muganga	examination,medical Assessment or evaluation.
igipimo c'amaso	eye test Catch all phrase for ophthalmologic examination.
igipimo c'amatwi	hearing test Audiologic evaluation.
igipimu cumuti ushobora kwica	lethal dose The amount of a drug required to cause death.
igisaga	excess Surplus or overabundance.
igisambo	hyperphagia Excessive food ingestion.
igise	childbirth Parturition; the process of labor and delivery of an infant.
igisebe kivuye kuguturirwa namazi ashushe cane	scald A burn injury from extremely hot water.

Kirundi	English
igishato c'ugutwi	earlobe The soft, fleshy inferior portion of the pinna.
igisibo	absence of
igisigo	constipation A condition exhibited by difficulty in having a bowel movement due to hard stools.
igitabiza	pancreas A gland that secretes digestive enzymes into the duodenum and insulin and glucagon into the blood.
igitangu (ifumberi)	deer tick Ixodes scapularis.
igitangurirwa	spider
igitangurirwa kinini	tarantula A large hairy spider found mainly in the tropics.
igitebo	stretcher A device used to carry a patient in the supine position.
igitega	flat Level or even; without bulges.
igitigu	liver A large glandular organ in the right upper quadrant that functions in digestive processes, as well as, neutralizing toxins.
igitobozi	drill Cylindrical metal tool uses for creating a hole in bone in surgery.
igitsina	sex Gender.
igitsintsiri	calcaneus Commonly called the heel bone.
igitsintsiri	heel Proximal portion of the plantar aspect of the foot.
igituba	vagina The canal in a female that extends from the vulva to the cervix.
igituntu	tuberculosis Any infectious disease caused by Mycobacterium.
igufa	bone Skeletal tissue formed by osteoblasts.
igufa inini ry'inkokera	ulna The smaller bone in the forearm.
igufa ro mumusaya, rir inyuma y ugutwi	mastoid Referring to the mastoid process.
igufa ryaboze	sequestrum Necrotic bone present in an injured or diseased bone.
igufa ryuruti rwumugongo	vertebra A term for each bone surrounding the spine.
igufa ry'igisigati	cartilage Firm, relatively non-vascular connective tissue.
igufa ry'ikiwuno	coccyx The small bone formed by the natural fusion of rudimentary vertebrae.
igufa ry'ikiwuno	ilium The large bone at the superior aspect of the pelvis which is present bilaterally.
igufa ry'itako; umuwero	femur The long bone in the thigh.
Igufa rzo mu gikonjo	cuneiform The three bones between the navicular bone and the metatarsals.
igwirirana ry amazi mudusaho twubwonko	hydrocephalus The excessive accumulation of cerebral spinal fluid in the brain causing enlargement of the head.
igwirirana ry amazi mugikiriza	hydrothorax Accumulation of fluid within the thoracic cavity.
ihagarara ry'umutima	cardiac arrest Cessation of function of the heart.
ihaha	lung One of a pair of respiratory organs.
ihasi	twins Two infants born at the same birthing.(identical twins)
ihere	scabies A skin condition exhibited by intense pruritus and a macular rash commonly in the perineal and interdigital spaces.

Kirundi	English
iherezo	end point The last stage of a process.
iherezo ryo kuvugra	disease outcome The response obtained from treatment.
ihigimba cumbwonko	subdural The area between the dura mater and the arachnoid membrane.
ihindagana	pallor Unusually pale appearance.
ihinduka	alteration The process of change or modification.
Ihingurwa ry amaraso	hemopoiesis The production of blood cells from stem cells.
ihingurwa ry intanga	spermatogenesis The production of spermatozoa.
ihotorwa ryamara	volvulus Twisting of the bowel leading to obstruction and sometimes perforation.
ihungabana	disequilibrium The absence of stability.
ihuriro	affinity To have a natural liking for.
ihuriro	appointment A previously scheduled time to see a person.
ihuriro ry imitsi mu kuboko	brachial plexus A cluster of nerves coming off the last four cervical and first thoracic spinal nerves form the nerve supply the the chest and arms.
ihusha	deviation Away from the norm.
ijigo	molar tooth Any of the most posterior teeth bilaterally which includes 8 deciduous and usually 12 permanent teeth.
ijisho bwigufa	tuberosity A protuberance. For instance the iliac tuberosity is a prominence on the surface of the ilium.
ijisho ry'ikirenge; urwambariro	ankle The area of the ankle joint.
ijwi	sound Vibrations that travel through air and are heard when reaching the ears.
ijwi	voice The sound produced through the larynx and out the mouth.
ikanzu	gown A sterile gown used during surgical procedures.
ikarabo	basin A small bowl used for washing.
ikarisiyumu	calcium A chemical element that is an essential component in teeth and bone.
ikibanza	site Location.
ikibengebenge (1)	radiation 1. The emission of energy in the form of electromagnetic waves. 2. Divergence from a common point.
ikibero	thigh The body region between the inguinal crease and knee.
ikibibi	birthmark A benign brown or red patch one is born with.
ikibugu	tsetse fly An insect that transmits the protozoa trypanosoma and can cause sleeping sickness.
ikicyaganuzi	calf, soreness or pain in the
ikida	obesity Having a body mass index over 30kilograms/meters squared.
ikidzjicyo cyera	sclera The white outer covering of the eyeball.
ikifukunyi	syncope Sudden loss of consciousness.
ikifundo	nodule A small node in the skin of up to 1cm and in the lung up to 3cm.
ikifunzi	fist When a person has their fingers clenched tightly to the palm.
ikigaga	congenital defect A disease or anomaly present from birth.
ikigagara	stretcher used to carry a corpse

135

Kirundi	English
ikigango	Achilles tendon Also called calcaneal tendon; tendon with insertion at the gastrocnemius & soleus into the tuberosity of the calcaneus
ikiganza	hand, palm of
ikiganza	palm The anterior aspect of the hand.
ikigohe	eyelid Palpebra.
ikigohegohe	eyebrow Supercilium.
ikigongogongo	sacrum The bone formed by five fused vertebrae that is situated between the two hip bones.
ikihazi	hernia An abnormal bulge of bowel through muscle.
ikihogohogo	larynx A hollow muscular structure that contains the vocal cords.
ikihoro	laceration An injury that is a cut/slice in the skin.
ikihura	vitiligo The appearance of non-pigmented white patches on otherwise normal skin; hair is usually white in the affected areas.
ikihute cy'ikituba	abscess, vulvar Collection of pus and swelling of the vulva.
ikikomere; ikisebe	injury A wound, abrasion or contusion.
ikimenyeco cindwara ya mburugu	rupia A sign of tertiary syphilis in which there are bullae or vesicles formed on the skin that erupt and form crusts.
ikimenyetso c'indwara	symptom A physical feature that is characteristic of disease.
ikimuga	cripple A person with a physical disability; not used in polite society.
ikinena; akusino	clitoris A small erectile body in the anterosuperior aspect of the vulva.
ikinini	capsule Medication in the form of a capsule.
ikinini co mugisusu	suppository A delivery system for medication placed in an orifice.
ikinogo	vagina, opening of the
ikinure	omentum A peritoneal fold passing from the stomach to another abdominal organ.
ikinutsi	ulcer A concave wound caused by a break in the integrity of skin or mucous membrane. (duodenal ulcer)
ikinutsi	wound A tissue injury of varying severity.
ikinyamwonga	shellfish An aquatic shelled crustacean or mollusk.
ikinyawashi	adenitis The inflammation of a gland.
ikinygishi	gum Gingiva.
ikiragi	deaf-mute Inability to hear or speak.
ikirangi	mute Refraining from or being speechless.
ikirato	shoe Article of clothing worn on each foot.
ikirato c'intoke	glove Covering for hand protection.
ikiremo cy'umwana; intutu	nappy Diaper
ikiremwa nyohabuzima	parasite An organism that lives on or within another organism without benefit to the latter.
ikirenge	foot (sole of the foot) The lower extremity distal to the ankle.
ikirenge cy'ukuguru	malleolus A bony protrusion on medial and lateral aspect of each ankle.
ikirenge gifyase	pes planus Medical term for flat foot.

Kirundi	English
ikirimba	fistula An abnormal communication between two organs or an organ and the skin, as in rectovaginal fistula.
ikirimba	furuncle A painful erythematous nodule with a central core.
ikiringo c'imyaka cumi	decade Ten years.
ikiriro	heart murmur An abnormal heart sound usually related to valvular disease.
ikiriyo	mourning A period of grieving.
ikiruhuko	rest Relaxation or respite.
ikirungurira	esophageal reflux Regurgitation of the stomach contents into the esophagus.
ikirungurira	heartburn Synonym of pyrosis.
ikirungurira	pyrosis Synonym for heartburn.
ikirungurira; iseseme	nausea A feeling that one wants to vomit.
ikirusu	hernia, epigastric Hernia through the linea alba superior to the navel.
ikisebe cy'ikiwere	breast abscess Pus collection in the breast.
ikisere	discharge, nasal Nasal secretions.
ikisero	nasal mucus Secretions coming from the nose.
ikiseru	coryza An acute condition exhibited by copious nasal discharge.
ikisheshwe	croup An acute laryngeal condition that is accompanied by a hoarse, barking cough.
ikishya	stitch Common term for a sharp pain under the breast.
ikisigo	colic Acute abdominal pain.
ikisigo	acne Inflamed or infected sebaceous glands.
ikisigo	gout Monosodium urate crystal deposition disease.
ikisigo	irritable bowel syndrome A gastrointestinal syndrome characterized by bloating, gas, constipation and diarrhea without an identified cause.
ikisumbano; ifufu	hematoma A mass containing blood.
ikivimbe	bubo An inflamed, swollen lymph node in the axilla or inguinal region.
ikivugwa	overt Not hidden.
ikivyeyi	urinary retention Inadequately emptying the bladder.
ikivyimba	lipoma A benign tumor consisting of fat cells.
ikivyimba	lymphoma A malignant disease of the lymph system, Hodgkin's lymphoma for example.
ikivyimba	malignancy Tendency of a tumor to invade normal tissue.
ikivyimba	mass Tumor.
ikivyimba	tumor A benign or malignant overgrowth of tissue.
ikivyimba co kurukoba canke mu mutima bivuye ku ndwara ya mburugu	gumma A soft granulomatous tumor of the skin or cardiovascular system seen in tertiary syphilis.
ikivyimba co mumavya	seminoma A malignant tumor of the testis.
ikiwuno	groin The genital region.
ikiwuwitsi	eschar Dry, hard, dead tissue commonly seen with a chronic pressure ulcer or anthrax.

137

Kirundi	English
ikiyiko kinini	teaspoon A measure instrument that holds 5 milliliters of fluid.
ikiyo	monitor A person that observes a process or a monitoring device.
ikiza	endemic When a disease is commonly found in a location or in a people group.
ikiza	epidemic Ubiquitous development of an infectious disease.
ikizeze; wugumye	obtuse Rather insensitive or hard to understand.
ikizigira	arm, upper
ikizigira	humerus The long bone in the upper arm.
ikizigira	upper limb Referring to either arm.
ikizimgami; uworohe	numbness Decreased sensation to tactile stimuli.
ikoreshwa ry impwemu kurugero runini	hyperbaric Use of gas at a higher than normal pressure.
ikura rirengeje urugero ry umushatsi	hypertrichosis Excessive hair growth.
ikwiragizwa	dissemination To be spread or dispersed widely.
ikyekezi	gumboil Swelling noted on the gingiva over a dental abscess.
imatera	mattress A fabric case filled with material, used for sleeping.
imbangwe	tourniquet A device tied tightly around an extremity to diminish blood flow or blood loss.
imbanyi iri inyuma y'igitereko	ectopic pregnancy A pregnancy that is not intrauterine.
imbaragasa	flea A small wingless insect that feeds on blood of mammals.
imbavu	side A position medial or lateral to center.
imbeba	rat A rodent that looks like a large mouse.
imbeba	rodent A gnawing mammal that includes rats and mice.
imbeho	algid cold
imbere	anterior Toward the front.
imbere	beforehand In advance or previously.
imbere	forwards Towards the front.
imbere mu	inside Inner part, center.
imbere y amavuko	antenatal Refers to events before birth.
imbere y ugutwi	preauricular Anterior to the ear.
imbere,	ventral Referring to the underside but in humans, a ventral hernia, for example, refers to an abdominal hernia.
imbonero	iris The anterior portion of the vascular tunic of the eye.
imbonero	pupil The opening at the center of the iris.
imbonero	lens The transparent chamber between the posterior chamber and the vitreous body.
imboro	penis Male genital organ used for the transfer of sperm and elimination of urine.
imbugita yo kubaga	scalpel A knife used during surgery for incision of skin and tissue.
Imbugita yo kwa muganga	bistoury; scalpel A surgical knife.
imbumbamubiri	vitamin
imburukutwi	ear, the area behind and below the
imbwa	cramp A painful contraction of muscles.

Kirundi	English
imetero yo gupima	tape measure A long length of tape, marked at intervals for measuring.
imeze nkinyuzi	filiform Threadlike.
Imibango	genu valgum A condition exhibited by the knees turning inward, commonly referred to as knock-knee.
imibembe	leprosy A contagious disease caused by Mycobacterium leprae that causes insensate papules and disfiguration.
imibeme	Hansen's disease Leprosy
Imicafu y umubiri	exudate The fluid, cells, and debris found in the tissues or a cavity (like pleural space) during inflammation.
Imigwi y ' amaraso ABO	ABO system The system using human blood antigens to determine blood type.
iminwa minini	macrocheilia Abnormally large lips.
imirero y'uwara	nail matrix or nail bed The area of the corium on which the nail rests.
imiringoti y indugu	bile ducts The structures that are conduits for passage of bile from the liver and gallbladder to the duodenum.
imisonga iza mumwanya wo gushukwa	priapism A painful and abnormally prolonged erection.
Imisonga mu kwikanira	dyschezia Pain experienced during defecation.
imisonga ya rimatizime	rheumatic pain Pain related to rheumatoid arthritis.
imisonga yo mu misoso	myalgia Muscle pain.
imisonga yo mugitereko	after-pains The pain experienced after childbirth caused by uterine contractions.
imisonga yo mukwezi	premenstrual syndrome A cluster of emotional, behavioral, and physical symptoms that occur in the premenstrual phase of the menstrual cycle and resolve with the onset of menstruation.
imisoso igize umubiri	motor Referring to muscles.
imisozi; umusozi	elephantiasis A condition caused by nematode parasites leading to lymphatic obstruction and limb or scrotal swelling.
imisuha	elephantiasis of the scrotum A condition caused by nematode parasites leading to lymphatic obstruction scrotal swelling.
imisuhuko	feel better or get better To have improved health symptomatically.
imisurusura	ligature A thread used to tie a vessel.
imisuzi	flatulence The gas expulsed from the anus.
imiti irwanya kuvura kwamaraso	anticoagulant Medication used to inhibit coagulation.
imiti y ibisahuzi	anticonvulsant Medication used to treat seizures.
imiti y ubushe bwumubiri	anti-inflammatory Medication used to reduce inflammation.
imiti yinzoka	anthelmintic An agent used to destroy worms.
imiti yo gucibwamo	anti-diarrheal Medication used to treat diarrhea.
imiti yo kkuyinga	antidepressant Medication used to treat depression.
imiti yo kuringaniza uruvyaro	oral contraceptive Tablet taken by mouth to prevent pregnancy.
imiti yo mu kanwa	oral medication Medicine taken by mouth.

Kirundi	English
imitisi yamaraso	vascular Referring to a blood vessel.
imitsi ifata inyama zo kumaguru	hamstrings Tendons of the posterior thigh.
imitsi yo kukuboko	muscle, biceps
imitsi yo kwitako	quadriceps The anterior thigh muscle composed of four muscles.
imitsi yo mugatuntu	muscle, intercostal
imitsi yo mumugongo	spinal cord The bundle of nerves that with the brain comprise the central nervous system.
imitsi yo munda	muscle, abdominal
imodoka itwara abagwaye; ambilansi	ambulance A vehicle that carries the sick or injured.
impande y amafyigo	perinephric Around the kidney.
impande zose	bilateral Referring to both sides.
impfuvyi	orphan A child without parents
impinduka yumuti	drug reaction Typically refers to an adverse effect of medication.
impindura	ileum The third portion of the small intestine, extending from the jejunum to the ileocecal valve.
impinyanyuro	adjustment A modification of a plan.
impumyi	blind person Person with absence of sight.
impungenge	vertigo A sensation of imbalance with many possible causes.
impwemu	air
impwemu	breath One respiration.
impwemu zikoreshwa muguhema neza	tidal volume The amount of air inspired with each breath. One can set a ventilator to deliver a preset number of milliliters of oxygenated air with each breath.
imudzi w'amaraso	vein A vessel carrying blood back toward the heart.
imurikwa ry ivyumba vyumutima canke vyubwonko	ventriculography Roentgenography of the ventricles after administration of contrast media.
Imvange, bivanze	heterogenous That which originates outside the organism.
imvugo	speech Oral articulation.
imvugo itarongorotse	inarticulate Indistinct speech.
imvune	fracture A broken bone.
imvune ukuboko	broken (arm) Fracture of the arm.
imyaka yo kubaho	life expectancy The length of time a person is anticipated to live.
inama	advice Recommendations regarding prudent further actions.
inambu	appetite A desire to eat.
inankunkuma	prepuce of clitoris The external skin fold of the labia minora which forms a cap over the clitoris.
incamake	compendium A concise summary about a subject.
incavyi	lump A protuberance.
ince	hymen A membrane in the vagina.
incuro umuntu ahema kumunota	respiratory rate The number of breaths per minute.
incuti	relation 1. A person who has a blood or marriage connection.

140

Kirundi	English
inda	abdomen The portion of the body bordered by the diaphragm and the pelvis.
inda	crab louse Phthirus pubis is formal name for a louse that infests pubic hair and causes intense itching.
inda	pregnancy The period of being pregnant.
inda haratotera	stomach cramps Sensation of muscle contraction in the epigastric area.
inda rikuze	gravida Pregnant woman.
inda; umushishito	stomach Organ of digestion between the esophagus and small bowel.
indaya	prostitute A person who exchanges goods or services for sex.
indihagizi	pulse The rhythmic throbbing of arteries felt at major vessels.
indihagizi y'umutima	flutter,atrial Used to describe a cardiac rhythm disturbance, as in atrial flutter.
indihaguzi	heart beat A single contraction of the heart.
indimwe	family
indorerezi	finger, extra Congenital 6th finger.
indrwara yo gukama amaraso	anemia Lower than normal red blood cell count.
indrwara y'ibubura ry'urukoba	dermatitis Non-specific inflammation of the skin.
Indugu	gallbladder The organ adjacent to the liver that stores bile and secretes it into the duodenum.
induru	groan A deep inarticulate sound made due to pain or despair.
indurwe	bile An alkaline fluid secreted by the liver to aid digestion.
indwaa yo gukama amosozi	xerophthalmia A manifestation of Vitamin A deficiency exhibited by dryness of the cornea and conjunctiva.
indwara	sickness Illness or a state of disease.
indwara	disease Malady or disorder.
indwara	illness Diseases, sickness or malady.
indwara bita leishmaniose	kala-azar A disease caused by Leishmania donovani that is exhibited by weight loss, fever, anemia and hepatosplenomegaly.
indwara idakira	terminal illness A disease with no viable treatment with death being inevitable.
indwara ifata amahuriro y'amagufwa	arthritis Joint inflammation.
indwara irenze urugero	acute Abrupt onset of disease.
indwara itazwi ikiyitera	idiopathic Relating to a disease with an unknown cause.
indwara iterwa no kurumwa n'inyamaswa	rabies An infectious viral disease transmitted through the bite of a mammal. Symptoms include hydrophobia, pharyngeal spasms and hyperactivity.
indwara mpuzabitsina	venereal disease A condition transmitted via sexual intercourse.
indwara y amabere	mastitis Inflammation of the breast.
indwara y amafzigo	nephritis A general term meaning inflammation of a kidney that is further categorized depending on the associated pathology.

Kirundi	English
indwara y amahaha	histoplasmosis A fungal pulmonary infection from bat and bird excrement.
indwara y amara	colitis Inflammation of the colon.
indwara y amara	megacolon Abnormal enlargement and dilatation of the colon.
indwara y amaso	blepharitis Inflammation of the eyelids.
Indwara y amaso	glaucoma A condition characterized by increased intraocular pressure.
indwara y amaso	ophthalmia Profound inflammation of the eye or its structures.
indwara y amaso	scleritis Inflammation of the eyeball.
indwara y amaso	trachoma An infection of the cornea and conjunctiva caused by Chlamydia.
indwara y amaso	catarrh Inflammation of a mucous membrane.
indwara y amatama	melitis Inflammation of the cheek.
indwara y amatwi	otitis Inflammation of the ear. (otitis media or otitis externa)
indwara y amatwi	otomycosis Fungal infection of the ear.

Kirundi	English
indwara y ibinyigishi	trench mouth Inflammation and ulceration of the gingivae.
indwara y icuririzi ifata mu maso, mubihimba vyirondoka, mu marasocanke munzara	thrush Candida albicans
indwara y igihogohogo	tracheitis Inflammation of the trachea.
indwara y ihinduka ryurukoba	port-wine mark Also called nevus flammeus, it is a vascular anomaly characterized by purplish skin discoloration.
indwara y imitsi	myositis Inflammation of muscle tissue.
Indwara y imitsi	deep vein thrombosis (DVT) A blood clot that forms within a vein, typically in the lower extremities.
indwara y imitsi nsoza bwenge	neuritis Inflammation of a nerve.
indwara y imitsi nsoza bwenge	neuropathy Structural of pathologic changes of the peripheral nervous system.
indwara y imitsi yo mumaso	risus sardonicus A spasm of the facial muscles causing what appears to be a smile on one's face.
indwara y indugu	cholecystitis Inflammation of the gallbladder.
indwara y inkovu	keloid Hypertrophic scar tissue that forms after a minor cut or surgical procedure.
indwara y inzaara	ingrown nail Also referred to as onychocryptosis.
indwara y inzoka	chigger A parasitic mite of the genus Trombicula.
indwara y iyinjira ry impemu mu mahaha	pneumothorax Abnormal presence of air between the lung and chest wall.
indwara y iyugagwa ry imitsi yamaraso yo mu bwonko	transient ischemic attack Cerebral ischemic changes resulting from transitory hypoperfusion.
Indwara y ubushuhe	sandfly fever A febrile illness transmitted by a sandfly, from the genus Phlebotomus, and found in the Mediterranean.
Indwara y ubushuhe ifatira kurukoba	tularemia An infectious disease caused by Francisella tularensis. The symptoms range from mild constitutional complaints to septic shock.
indwara y ubushuhe n umukozo utukura bivuye ku inyonko	blackwater fever A term used to describe the fever associated with malaria when the urine is reddish-black.
indwara y ubwonko buto	microcephalic A congenital deformity exhibited by an abnormally small head.
indwara y udusaho twumubiri tuvyimbishwa n amazi	hydrocele The accumulation of fluid in a body sac.
indwara y ukuvyimba mu kirenge	verruca A hyperplastic epidermal lesion, sometimes referred to as plantar wart.
indwara y umugongo	myelitis Inflammation of the spinal cord.
indwara y umukondo	omphalitis Inflammation of the umbilicus.
indwara y umutwe munini	macroencephaly Having an abnormally large head.
indwara y umwingo	Graves' disease A form of hyperthyroidism exhibited by a goiter and exophthalmos.
Indwara y urukoba	jock itch Pruritus caused by tinea cruris.
indwara y urukoba	hyperpigmentation, skin disease causing General term to describe skin darkening.

143

Kirundi	English
indwara y urukoba bita leishmaniose	**leishmaniasis** A condition caused by a flagellate protozoan parasite that is exhibited by visceral or dermatologic manifestations.
indwara y ururimi runini	**macroglossia** Abnormally large tongue.
indwara y uturingoti twamarira	**hordeolum** Inflammation of the sebaceous gland of the eye.
Indwara ya dengue	**dengue** A mosquito-borne viral disease exhibited by fever and joint pain.
Indwara ya iriseri yo mumushishito	**gastroduodenal ulcer** A lesion in the mucosal lining of the stomach or duodenum.
indwara ya Peyironi	**Peyronie's disease** Curvature of the penis during an erection due to plaque.
indwara yamafyigo	**renal failure** Diminution of kidney function.
Indwara yamahaha	**emphysema** Abnormal enlargement of the airspaces distal to the terminal bronchioles.
indwara yamaraso, afise mikorobe nyinshi	**septicemia** A systemic disease in which microorganisms or their toxins are in the blood stream.
indwara yigitereko gisohokera mu gisundi	**prolapse of the uterus** Eversion of the uterus through the vagina.
indwara yihotorwa ryivya	**testicular torsion** Rotation of the spermatic cord resulting in testicular ischemia.
indwara yikirimi	**uvulitis** Inflammation of the uvula.
indwara yimitsi (in kirundi, the tem imitsi has several meaning from different uses. It can be Vessels, Muscles, or tendons)	**tendinitis** Inflammation of a tendon.
indwara yo gufungura nabi	**kwashiorkor** A form of malnutrition from inadequate protein intake.
indwara yo gushuha	**rat bite fever** As the name implies, it is a condition exhibited by fever, nausea and skin erythema after one is bitten by a rat.
indwara yo gusinzira ijisho rimwe	**blepharospasm** A spasm of the orbicularis oculi muscle that causes closure of the eyelid.
indwara yo gusomana	**mononucleosis** An infectious disease exhibited by malaise and lymphadenopathy.
indwara yo guta umutwe	**psychosis** A profound mental disorder that can include delusions and hallucinations.
indwara yo ku kwuma kurukoba	**ichthyosis** A congenital anomaly exhibited by excessively dry, thick skin.
Indwara yo kubira ivyuya	**dyshidrosis** Dysregulation of sweating
indwara yo kubona ibintu bibiri mwijisho rinwe	**monodiplopia** Double vision in only one eye.
indwara yo kubora mubihimba vy amaso	**gonorrheal ophthalmia** An acute purulent conjunctivitis that can occur in neonates within 2-5 days of birth.
indwara yo kubura amaraso mumahaha	**pulmonary embolism** A sudden blockage of a lung artery frequently emanating from a blood clot in one's leg.
indwara yo kubura impwemu mwijoro	**sleep apnea** Episodic apnea during sleep that is exhibited by daytime symptoms of fatigue, difficulty concentrating and sleepiness.
indwara yo kudatandukanya amabara	**color blindness** The inability to distinguish colors.
indwara yo kufungua nabi	**marasmus** Progressive weight loss and emaciation.

Kirundi	English
indwara yo kugendagenda umuntu asinziriye	somnambulism Sleepwalking.
Indwara yo kugigimiza	dysphasia Difficulty in speaking caused by cerebral dysfunction.
indwara yo kugira ubwoba budasanzwe	panic attack Sudden, profound anxiety.
Indwara yo kumira	dysphagia Difficulty in swallowing.
indwara yo kunzara	onychia Inflammation of the toenail or fingernail matrix.
indwara yo kunzara	onychomycosis Fungal disease of the toenails or fingernails.
indwara yo kutasinzira (kutungara amaso)	lagophthalmos Characterized by the inability to close the eyelid completely over the eye.
indwara yo kutibagira	hypermnesia Unusually good memory.
indwara yo kutumva akanovera	gustatory agnosia The loss of the sense of taste.
indwara yo kutumva neza	auditory agnosia Caused by a temporal lobe lesion, it is characterized by inability to recognize sounds as words.
Indwara yo kuva amaraso mumaso	hemophthalmia Bleeding within the eye.
Indwara yo kuva amaraso mumubiri	hemophilia A hereditary bleeding disorder characterized by hemarthroses and deep tissue bleeding as a result of absence of a coagulation factor such as factor VIII.
indwara yo kuvyimba amabere	gynecomastia Enlargement of the breasts.
indwara yo kuvyimba ibinyigishi; ividzjegezi	gingivitis Inflammation of the gums.
Indwara yo kuvyimba ukuguru bita Erysipele mukinofunofu	erysipelas An acute infection caused by Streptococcus pyogenes that causes fever along with swelling and inflammation. The infection frequently effects the face or one leg.
indwara yo kwifata nabi	behavior disorder An abnormal mental state.
indwara yo kwikanga	hallucination A perception that is not based on reality.
indwara yo kwisobako	urinary incontinence Involuntary micturition.
indwara yo kwisobako usinziriye	enuresis Involuntary urination.
indwara yo kwuma urukoba	xerosis Pathological dryness of the skin or mucous membranes.
indwara yo kwuzura amazi mumahaha	pulmonary edema Characterized by abnormal fluid buildup in the lungs.
Indwara yo mu bishinyi	gingival Referring to the gums.
indwara yo mu bwonko	mad cow disease Bovine spongiform encephalopathy, a disease that cause cerebral degeneration exhibited by ataxia.
indwara yo mu kirenge	athlete's foot Common term for tinea pedis.
indwara yo mu mutwe ikurikira kwibaruka	post-partum depression Depressed mood occurring after childbirth.
indwara yo mu nzanyi	balanitis Inflammation of the glans of the penis.
indwara yo mubihimba vy rondoka	pelvic inflammatory disease Generally a bacterial infection affecting a women with potential involvement of the uterus, fallopian tubes, ovaries and cervix.
indwara yo mubihimba vyirondoka	venereal wart Common term for condyloma acuminatum.

Kirundi	English
indwara yo muduheha dutwara imbuto mugitereko kumugore	salpingitis Inflammation of the fallopian tubes.
indwara yo mugisusu	proctitis Inflammation of the rectum.
Indwara yo mukayiba kinda	cystitis Inflammation of the urinary bladder.
indwara yo mumagage	laryngospasm Sudden, involuntary muscle contraction of the larynx.
indwara yo mumara	enteritis Inflammation of the intestines.
Indwara yo mumatwi	ear infection General term referring to otitis media or otitis externa.
indwara yo mumazuru	rhinitis A viral infection or allergic reaction exhibited by nasal mucosal inflammation.
indwara yo mumuhogo	esophagitis Inflammation of the esophagus.
indwara yo mumutwe	schizophrenia A chronic mental condition exhibited by delusions, hallucinations, and faulty perception.
indwara yo mumutwe iterwa no guhagarika inzoga bukwi na bukwi	delirium tremens A condition seen when alcohol is withdrawn which is exhibited by restlessness, hallucinations and tremors.
indwara yo mumutwe ituma umuntu yemeza ibitarivyo	delusion A belief that is contradictory to rational thought.
Indwara yo mumutwe ivuye mu kuborerwa canke kufata imiti myinshi	dual diagnosis Term used to describe the presence of alcohol/drug addiction associated with a psychiatric diagnosis such as depression.
indwara yo munda iterwa no kudya inyama yapfuye	trichinosis A disease caused by meat infected by Trichinella spiralis causing fever and gastrointestinal effects.
Indwara yo mungingo	gonorrheal arthritis A type of arthritis caused by the gram negative diplococcus Neisseria gonorrhoeae.
indwara yo murutugu	frozen shoulder Common term for adhesive capsulitis.
indwara yomumutwe yinyuma yo kwibaruka	post-partum psychosis A episode of abnormal thought or hallucinations following delivery.
indwara yubushuhe	Rift valley fever A human febrile illness that is an endemic disease in sheep, transmitted by mosquitos and direct contact and caused by a virus of the family Bunyaviridae.
indwara yubushuhe	scarlet fever A condition caused by streptococci that is exhibited by fever and a bright red (scarlet) rash.
indwara yuduce twamahaha	bronchitis Inflammation of the mucous membranes of the bronchioles that causes bronchospasm and cough.
indwara yumugongo	scoliosis A lateral curvature of the spine.
indwara yumuringoti nsozantaga	urethritis Inflammation of the urethra.
indwara yumutima	pericardial tamponade Decrease in systemic perfusion related to a collection of fluid in the pericardial space.
indwara yurukoba	impetigo
Indwara yurukoba	ecchymosis Skin discoloration caused by bleeding beneath the epidermis.
indwara yurukoba iterwa nudukoko	hives Urticaria
indwara yuturingoti twumukoyo	ureteritis Inflammation of the ureter.
indwara y'amabavu	pemphigus A skin disorder with large bullous lesions.
indwara y'amara n'inda	gastroenteritis A bacterial or viral infection that leads to vomiting and diarrhea.

146

Kirundi	English
indwara y'amaso iterwa n'ubusaza	presbyopia Farsightedness associated with aging.
indwara y'igisukari	diabetes mellitus A disease exhibited by a deficiency of the pancreatic hormone insulin.
indwara y'igitigu (ingwara y'igitigu y'umugera wo mu murwi B)	hepatitis Inflammation of the liver. (hepatitis B)
indwara y'ikiza gikwiye hose	pandemic When a disease is present over an entire region.
indwara y'uburima	dandruff Dead skin found in the hair.
indwara y'uburima	favus Tinea capitis caused by Trichopyton schoenleini.
indwara y'uburima	tinea capitis Ringworm of the scalp, a fungal infection.
indwara y'umushihito	gastritis Inflammation of the stomach.
indwara y'umutima	heart disease Generic term generally meant to imply coronary disease.
indwara y'urwiba	amnesia The inability to remember past events.
indwara zibikoko zandukira abantu	zoonosis An animal-born disease that can be transmitted to humans, such as rabies.
indwara zivyuririzi	pneumocystis jiroveci pneumonia. A pulmonary infection associated with AIDS. Formerly called pneumocystis carinii pneumonia
indwara zo kumubiri	macula solaris Formal medical term describing a freckle.
indwara zo mu bihimba vy'irondoka	sexually transmitted disease (STD) A condition one obtains from another during sexual relations.
indwara zo mu matwi	otitis externa Inflammation of the middle ear
indwara zo mubihimba vyirondoka	genital herpes A sexually transmitted infection caused by herpes simplex.
Indwara zuturingoti dutwara amosozi	dacryocystitis Inflammation of a lacrimal sac.
Indwaraa yo munda ifata amara, urwagasha, n amahaha	cystic fibrosis A congenital disorder exhibited by abnormal thick mucous which leads to problems in the intestines, pancreas and lungs.
indwarayo mumuzi windyinyo	pulpitis Dental pulp inflammation.
indwarayumutima	pericarditis Inflammation of the pericardium.
indya	food Nutrition.
ingabirano	aptitude A natural talent for something.
ingaburo	diet The kinds of food a person eats.
inganga	ascaricide Agent that destroys ascaris.
ingeso	habit A custom or inclination.
ingingo	phalanges The long bones of the fingers or toes.
ingingo y'urutoke	knuckles Metacarpophalangeal joints or finger joints when the fist is closed.
ingingo; urugingo	joint Articulation of two adjacent bones.
ingohe	palpebra, palpebrae Eyelid, eyelids.
ingohe	cilia The hairs growing on the eyelid or a motile extension of a cell surface.
ingoma y ugutwi	ear-drum Common term for tympanic membrane.
ingoma y ugutwi	tympanic membrane The membrane between the external and middle ear.

147

Kirundi	English
ingorane	problem Difficulty or complaint.
ingorane zo mu mubiri	disorder Impairment.
ingovyi	afterbirth The tissue expelled after the birth of a child that includes the placenta and allied membranes.
ingovyi izibira umwana	placenta praevia A condition in which the placenta covers the cervical os.
ingovyi yahomotse	placental abruption Premature detachment of a normally situated placenta.
inguge	cynocephaly Craniostenosis in which the cranium slopes back from the orbits.
inguvu	potency Strength or power.
inkabuzo	enzyme A compound that acts as a catalyst for reactions within cells as assists with digestion outside of cells.
inkabuzo	histamine A chemical responsible for the reaction exhibited when a person has an allergic reaction.
Inkabuzo yo mu rwagasha	glucagon A pancreatic enzyme responsible for breakdown of glycogen to glucose.
Inkabuzo yo mu rwagasha	insulin A hormone produced by the pancreas and synthetically to control blood glucose levels.
inkabuzo zigize amaraso	hemoglobin An iron containing protein used for the transport of oxygen in blood.
inkaka	ureter The conduit between each kidney and the urinary bladder.
inkavyi	head contusion, resulting in a superficial hematoma
inkecuru	hangnail A loose piece of skin attached near the medial or lateral nail fold.
inkikuro	circumference The distance around an object or part.
inkingi y'ururimi	frenulum linguae A fold of tissue extending from the floor of the mouth to the midline of the under part of the tongue.
inkokora	olecranon The bony protrusion at the proximal ulna at the elbow.
inkokora; nyamanyakawiri	elbow The joint between the humerus and radius/ulna.(right elbow, left elbow)
inkomezi	strength Force, might or vigor.
inkoni yo kwishimikiza	cane Device used to aid walking (walking stick).
inkoro; igufa ry'ikikaraza	sternum Commonly called the breast bone, it consists of the corpus, manubrium and xiphoid process.
inkorora	cough Forceful expulsion of air from the lungs.
Inkorora yagahehera	dry cough A cough without sputum production.
inkorora y'akanira	pertussis Synonym for whooping cough.
inkorora y'akanira	whooping cough Pertussis
inkovu	scar The fibrotic tissue that forms at the site of a wound.
inkovu ivyimvye	fibrosis Connective tissue that is scarred and thickened after injury.
inkukura	erosion The gradual destruction of surface tissue.
inkumi (umusore)	single woman (single man) Not married.
inkungugu	dust Dry earthen particles found on the ground and surfaces.

Kirundi	English
inkurikizi	sequela A medical problem related to an initial injury or disease.(late sequelae)
inkurikizi	side effect An expected but unwanted effect of a medication.
inkurikizi y imiti	iatrogenic A problem caused by medical treatment.
inkurikizi zimiti	adverse effect In reference to medication use, it is an undesirable consequence of the drug.
inkurikizi zo guhahamuka; indwara nyakuri	post-traumatic stress syndrome (PTSD)
Inndwara y urwagasha	pancreatitis Inflammation of the pancreas.
ino	toe Any of the digits of of the feet.
ino rinini	toe, big First digit of the foot.
inshinge bita "depo-vera injections"	depo-vera injection A birth control medication injected every three months.
insiguro y indwara	pathogenesis The course of a disease.
insondo	aggression Violent or hostile behavior.
intambwe	pace Consistent and continuous movement.
intambwe ishimishije	milestone An event indicative of a certain stage of development.
intambwe yanyuma	end stage Terminal stage. End stage cancer means there is no cure possible and death is imminent.
intandara	epilepsy A condition associated with abnormal brain activity and exhibited by sudden, recurrent convulsions, sensory disturbances and loss of consciousness.
Intandara zabagore bibungenze	eclampsia A maternal condition characterized by convulsions and hypertension that can lead to maternal and fetal death.
intanga	semen
intanga	sperm Short term for spermatozoon.
intanga; igitereko	uterus The hollow organ in the female pelvis where a fertilized ovum embeds and grows.
intanguro y indwara	presenting symptom The initial subjective complaint that initiated a visit.
intantu	pubis The anterior inferior part of the hip bone on each side that articulates at the pubic symphysis.
intebe bicarako mu koga	shower chair A seating device one sits on while showering.
intebe yo gusunika umugwayi	wheelchair A wheeled device used for propulsion.
integabiza	supplies Stock or reserves.
intege	calf Muscles of the posterior portion of the lower leg.
intege	lymph node An area of organized lymphatic tissue.
intege nke y' imidzi	muscle weakness Decreased muscular function.
intenga y'umuwiri	torso The trunk of the body.
intera y'umutwe	parietal bone The bone on either side of the vault of the cranium.
intera y'umutwe	vertex The crown of the head.
intimba	grief Deep sorrow.
intoboro	fossa A shallow depression.
Intoboro yigufa	foramen An opening in a bone.
Intoboro yigufa ryo mumutwe	foramen magnum The hole in the skull that the spinal cord passes through.

149

Kirundi	English
intoboro y'ijisho	orbit The bony structure enclosing the eyeball.
intoke ndende	arachnodactyly A condition exhibited by abnormally long and slender fingers.
intoke ndende	macrodactyly Abnormally large digits.
intoke nyinshi	polydactyly Congenital anomaly exhibited by more than 5 digits on the hands and/or feet.
intonyanga	drop A single bit of fluid as in a drop seen while giving IV fluids.
intumbero	target An objective towards which efforts are directed.
intunganyakaronda	gene A unit of heredity that is passed on from parent to child.
intuntu	melancholia Profound sadness.
inyama	muscle A band if fibrous tissue that can contract.
inyama igize imitsi yo munda	fascia The fibrous sheath enclosing a muscle or organ.
Inyama itandukanya amaha no munda	diaphragm The muscular separation between the thoracic and abdominal cavities.
inyama iwoze	gangrene Tissue death from either impaired blood flow or an infection.
inyama yo mungingo y amagufa	meniscus A thin cartilage between joint surfaces.
inyama yo mwiteraniro ryurutugu	rotator cuff The structure around the capsule of the shoulder joint formed by the infraspinatus, supraspinatus, teres minor and subscapularis muscles.
inyama y'imidzimidzi	ligament A band of fibrous connective tissue that connects two bones or cartilage.
inyankane	allergy An immune response by the body to a compound it is hypersensitive to.
inyenzi	cockroach A beetle-like insect with long legs and antennae.
inyishu	reaction A response to an action.
inyishu zibipimo	lab result The data obtained from a laboratory test.
inyo	anus The body opening distal to the rectum.
inyondwi	tick
inyonko	malaria A condition caused by a protozoan of the genus Plasmodium. It is transmitted by mosquitos and is exhibited by fever, chills, headache. In the severe form it can lead to convulsions, increased ICP and death.
inyonko; umururumbo	fever A temperature above the normal range.
inyonzo	hunchback Synonym of kyphosis.
inyonzo	kyphosis Abnormal outward curvature of the spine.
inyota	thirst The desire to drink.
inyota nyinshi	polydipsia Profound thirst.
inyubakaambubiri	protein A class of nitrogenous organic compound.
inyuma	after The time following an event.
inzahabu	gold Precious metal with atomic number of 79.
inzara	hunger A sense of discomfort caused by a lack of food.
inzina ry'umuryango	surname One's given "last" name that generally changes for women upon marriage to that of the man's surname.
inzira igomorora amaraso canke amazi yo mumubiri	shunt An alternate path for blood or fluid.
inzoga	alcohol Ethanol or ethyl alcohol.

Kirundi	English
inzoga (urwarwa)	beer A form of fermented alcohol. (banana beer)
inzoka	worm Any of long, slender, legless, soft-bodied invertebrates.
Inzoka yo kurukoba	guinea worm A parasitic nematode worm that, in cases of infection, lives under the skin, formally called Dracunculus medinensis.
inzoka yo mu gitigu	fluke Parasitic nematode worm; an example is Schistosoma.
inzoka yo munda	ascaris A nematode from genus intestinal lumbricoid parasite, also called round worm.
Inzoka yo munda	giardiasis A flagellate protozoa, Giardia lamblia, that causes diarrhea.
inzoka yo umubiri	pinworm Common term for Enterobius vermincularis; a nematode worm that is a parasite.
inzoka zo munda	nematode An endoparasite belonging to the class of the Nemathelminthes including roundworms and threadworms.
inzoka; ikiyoka	snake (snake venom)
inzozi	dream The thoughts or images occurring during sleep.
inzya	pubic hair Hair present in the perineal area.
in'ingoga	brisk Rapid or fast.
ipampa	cotton wool Raw cotton.
ipansuma yo guhagarika kuva amaraso	pressure dressing A dressing used for compression to reduce bleeding.
ipansuma yo ku nzanyi	bandage tied to a circumcised penis
ipasuka ry imiringoti itwara amaraso mu bwonko	apoplexy Extravasation of blood within an organ. For example, neonatal apoplexy is consistent with intracranial hemorrhage.
ipfundo	knot A fastening made by tying a suture, for instance.
ipfunywa ry imitsi yo kukirenge	carpopedal spasm A spasm of the carpus and the foot.
ipuderi	powder Fine dry particles.
iradiyo	x-ray
irekwe	hypersalivation Abnormal increase in salivation.
iriseri yumushishito	stomach ulcer Gastric ulcer.
iromba	exomphalos Umbilical hernia.
iromba	hernia, umbilical Protrusion of abdominal contents at the umbilicus.
irondo	hernia, inguinal Protrusion of abdominal-cavity contents through the inguinal canal.
iryinyo	tooth One of a set of hard, bony enamel coated structure in the jaw.
isabukuru y'amavuka	date of birth
isabuni	soap A compound made with fats/oils and an alkali; it is used for washing.
isaho nkingiramara	peritoneum The serous membrane covering the abdominal organs and lining the abdominal walls.
isaho y'umutima	pericardium The structure enclosing the heart which contains a fibrous outer layer and serous inner layer.
isari	starvation Death related to starvation.
isevu	hiccup Involuntary spasm of the diaphragm with sudden closure of the glottis; this causes a characteristic cough.

Kirundi	English
ishashara	candle A cylindrical piece of wax with a central wick.
ishimikiro	standing Position or status.
ishinyo	teeth, front The two maxillary teeth most anterior in the mouth.
Ishirahamwe Mpuzamakungu ry Amagara y Abantu.	World Health Organization (WHO)
ishuka	sheet (bed) A rectangular fabric covering a bed.
isi	mycosis A disease caused by a fungal infection.
isima	plaster cast Use of gypsum impregnated gauze to immobilize fractured extremities.
isima bashira ku mvune	cast; plaster cast Use of plaster of paris to immobilize an extremity.
isimbagurika ry umutima	arrhythmia An abnormal heart rhythm.
isimbasimba	gallop An abnormal heart sound.
isobero ryabagabo	urinal Device used by men to void while in bed or sitting.
Isohoka ry Ingovyi	expulsion of placenta Passage of the placenta out the cervix after childbirth.
Isohoka ry umukoyo	diuresis Increased excretion of urine.
isohoka ryuruzogi imbanyi itaravuka	prolapse of the umbilical cord Refers to the umbilical cord protruding from the cervix during active labor.
isohoro	iliopsoas A group of muscles inserting on the anterior aspect of the lesser trochanter of the femur.
isubirizwa	displacement Movement from normal position.
isukari	sugar A sweet crystalline substance made from a plant such as sugar cane.
isukari nyinshi mu mubiri	hyperglycemia Higher than normal level of glucose in the blood.
isuku	hygiene Practices related to cleanliness.
isumbi	lymphangitis Inflammation of the lymph vessels.
Isumbi	adenopathy Generally referring to a condition of the lymphatic glands.
isuna	foot and mouth disease A contagious viral disease exhibited by oral and digital vesicles.
isunikwa ry'ivyinjijwe mu mara	peristalsis The contractile action of the bowel.
isununu	nevus A benign, well-circumscribed growth of tissue of congenital origin.
isununu	wart A flesh colored growth that is also called verruca.
isununu mu ntantu	genital wart The common term for Condylomata acuminata.
Isura	general appearance The overall look of a patient.
isuzuma	assessment An medical evaluation.
isya ry'imfungurwa mu nda	digestion The process of enzymatic breakdown of food in the alimentary canal.
itako	hollow An indentation.
itako ry icuma	hip replacement Both joint surfaces are replaced by high density material such as plastic or metal.
itama	buccal Referring to the cheek.
itama	cheek Lateral facial tissue.
Itariki imiti iyopfirako	expiration date The date when a medication should no longer be used.

Kirundi	English
Itariki yo kwinjira mubitaro	date of admission Beginning date of hospitalization.
itaro irasa n'urufu	lethargy Absence of energy.
itengatwa	testicle One of a pair of organs in the male scrotum that produces sperm.
itera ryimitsi y amaraso yo kukirenge	dorsalis pedis pulse Pulse on dorsum of the foot.
itera ryumutima mu rudubi	ventricular fibrillation Chaotic and ineffective ventricular contractions.
itiro	asleep To be in a dormant or inactive state.
itori	sleep A nap or a snooze. (deep sleep)
ivi	knee The joint at the distal femur and proximal tibia.
ividzjekecyo	toothache Dental pain.
ivubi	wasp Any one of a winged hymenopterous insects.
ivuka	birth The process of bearing offspring from the uterus.
Ivunika ryamagufa yabana	fracture, greenstick A spiral fracture.
ivuriro	clinic A building where patients are evaluated.
ivuriro rito	health center A physical location where patients are treated.
ivyarementanijwe	confabulation The fabrication of experiences to compensate for memory loss.
ivyihutirwa cane	emergency An urgent, life-threatening situation.
ivyimba ry imiringoti itwara amaraso	arteriosclerosis Hardening and thickening of arterial walls.
ivyimba ry imitsi itwara amaraso mumavya	varicocele A cluster of varicose veins in the scrotum.
ivyimba ry'agasaho k'umusenyi k'urusogi	appendicitis Inflammation of the appendix.
ivyimba ry'umuhogo	laryngitis Inflammation of the larynx.
ivyinjijwe mu mubiri	food intake Quantitative record of nutritional intake.
ivyinjijwe mu mubiri amazi	fluid intake The amount of oral consumption plus the amount of intravenous fluids administered.
ivyirori; amarori	eyeglasses Eye wear used for cosmetic or prescription purposes.
ivyitezwe mu bipimo vy'indwara	prognosis The likely course of a disease.
ivyongewe	increment An increase on a fixed scale.
iwuye ry'isare	nephrolithiasis A calculus in the kidney.
iyaguka ryimitsi itwara amaraso	vasodilatation The process of making the blood vessels larger which decreases blood pressure.
iyicara ry umwana	fetal position Refers to how the fetus lies within the uterus.
Iyindi ndwara yishoboka	differential diagnosis A list of possible alternative diagnoses for a patient who is ill.
iyomviro	auditory canal, external Also called the external acoustic meatus; it leads from the auricle to the tympanic membrane.
iyugarwa ryimitsi yamaraso	vasoconstriction The process of making the blood vessels smaller which increases blood pressure.
iza	best Optimal or ideal.
izabana	eczema A medical condition exhibited by pruritic, red, scaly patches on the scalp, cheeks and extensor surfaces.
izina	name A word by which a person is known.

Kirundi	English
izjwi	vocal cords Paired folds of mucous membranes stretched across the larynx.
izosi	neck The part of the body that connects the body to the head.
izuru	nose The midface protuberance used for smelling and breathing.
kabiri	double Twice the size, quantity or strength.
kabiri	two times One action being done on two occasions.
kandi	also In addition.
kanseri	cancer; carcinoma A disease of uncontrolled abnormal cell growth.
kanseri	melanoma Malignant cancer, typically found in the skin.
kanseri y urukoba	Kaposi sarcoma Typically seen in AIDS patients, it is characterized by cutaneous reddish-purple macules and plaques.Also called multiple idiopathic hemorrhagic sarcoma.
kanzuya	minute Something very small.
karu	acid Substance with a pH less than 7.
kiba intabwe ku yindi	progressive Developing gradually.
kibangamye	life-threatening Potentially fatal.
kibangamye cane	insidious A slow, gradual and harmful advancement.
kibomvye	moist Damp or humid.
kiboneka cane	currently Presently.
kidadera	chronic When referring to an illness, it means recurring or persistent.
kigaragara	empty Containing nothing.
kigaragara	evident Obvious.
kigenda ciyongera	cumulative effect A consequence of successive additions.
kigumye	firm Hard or unyielding.
kigumye	hard Rigid or very firm.
kijanye no gutakaza amazi mu mubiri kubera ugusoba cane	diuretic Medication which causes an increased excretion of urine.
kijanye n'amabere	mammary Referring to the breast.
kijanye n'amagufa y'amano	metatarsal Referring to any of the metatarsal bones.
kijanye n'amagufa y'ikiganza	metacarpophalangeal Referring to the metacarpus and the phalanges.
kijanye n'amenyo	dental Referring to teeth.
kijanye n'inkingiramubiri	immune Being resistant to an infection.
kijanye n'umurizo	caudal Referring to a cauda.
kijanye n'umushishito	gastric Referring to the stomach.
kijanye n'umutwe	cephalic Towards the head.
kijanye n'uruhanga	frontal Referring to the anterior aspect, as in frontal lobe.
kijanye 'umugongo	dorsal Referring to the back or back surface.
kijugumira	palsy Paralysis that is usually associated with tremors.
kimenyerewe	usual Typical or normal.
kimputo	recurrent fever Repeated fever from an unknown cause.
kimputo	relapsing fever A recurrent bacterial infection, with fever, caused by Spirochetes.

Kirundi	English
kimputo	tick-borne fever A relapsing fever caused by a spirochete of the genus Borrelia.
kimwe	single Only one.
kimwenakimwe	upright Vertical or standing.
kinanye n'amahaha	pulmonary Referring to the lungs.
kinini cane	enormous Very large.
kinyaruka	quickening Signs of life noted by a mother as the fetus moves.
kinyegeye	discrete Separate and distinct.
kiregarega	loose Not tight.
kirekire cana rwose	giant Huge or massive.
kiremeye	heavy Possessing great weight.
kirenduka	viscous Having a thick, sticky consistency.
kitababaza	painless Not painful.
kitagira ico gifasha	irrelevant Not pertinent.
kitameze nk'ibindi	atypical Not usual.
kitanyengetera	impervious Not affected by.
kitaragera	premature Occurring earlier than expected.
kitarico namba	aberrant Different than normal.
kitazwi	unknown Uncertain or undisclosed.
kitera ingaruka mbi	detrimental Harmful.
kitica	harmless Safe or benign.
kitihutirwa	elective Non-urgent and not life-saving.
kitumvikana	incoherent Absence of intelligible speech.
kitumvikana	meaningless Having no significance.
kizunguzungu	giddiness A tendency to fall or dizziness.
kizwi hose	general Common or expected.
korera	cholera An infectious disease exhibited by vomiting and diarrhea and caused by Vibrio cholerae.
ku tetemera uruhande rumwe	monoplegia Paralysis of a single limb.
kuba ibisanzwe	common, to be That which is usual.
kuba maso	alert, to be Being in a watchful, ready state.
kuba maso	conscious Being award and being able to respond to one's surroundings.
kuba umuja ibyobezabwenge	drug dependence Addiction to a substance.
kubabara	suffer, to To be affected by an illness or sickness.
kubabara mukukira	odynophagia Pain associated with swallowing.
Kubabwa kumukoyo	dysuria Difficulty or pain upon urination.
kubaga akamirampeke	pallidectomy Surgical resection of all or part of the palate.
kubaga amafyigo	nephrotomy Surgical incision of the kidney.
kubaga amara	colectomy Surgical removal of part of the colon.
Kubaga amara	enterectomy Surgical resection of part of the intestine.
kubaga bagasubiriza igice kibonerana co mujisho	corneal transplant Surgical replacement of a cornea with a donor cornea.
kubaga ibere	mastectomy Surgical resection of one or both breasts.
kubaga ibisebe vyo kurukoba	exfoliation The shedding of scales.

155

Kirundi	English
kubaga ifyigo	nephrectomy Surgical removal of a kidney.
kubaga igihogohogo	tracheostomy Creation of a surgical opening in the trachea so a tube could be placed in the trachea.
kubaga igitereko	hysterectomy Surgical removal of the uterus.
kubaga igititgu	hepatectomy Partial or complete surgical resection of the liver.
kubaga igufa	osteotomy Creation of a surgical opening in bone.
kubaga ihaha	pneumonectomy Surgical excision of all or part of a lung.
kubaga indugu	cholecystectomy Surgical excision of the gallbladder.
kubaga irwagasha	pancreatectomy Surgical excision of part or all of the pancreas.
kubaga ivi	patellectomy Surgical excision of the patella.
kubaga ivya	orchidectomy Synonym of orchiectomy; removal of one or both testes.
kubaga kumuhogo	laryngotomy Surgical creation of an opening in the larynx.
kubaga mugikiriza	thoracotomy Surgical incision of the thorax.
kubaga mumaso	sclerotomy Surgical incision of the sclera.
kubaga mumazuru	rhinoplasty Plastic surgery performed on the nose.
kubaga mumuhogo	laryngectomy Surgical removal of the larynx.
Kubaga munda	laparotomy A surgical incision of the abdomen.
Kubaga munda	exploratory laparotomy Abdominal surgery with the intent of examining the abdominal contents.
kubaga prostate	prostatectomy Surgical excision of the prostate.
kubaga ubwonko canke uruti rw umugongo	neurosurgery Surgery of the brain or spinal cord.
Kubaga umuhogo	esophagectomy Surgical removal of the esophagus.
kubaga umushishito	gastrostomy A surgical creation of an opening in the stomach.
Kubaga umushishito	gastrectomy Complete or partial surgical resection of the stomach.
Kubaga umusipa	herniorrhaphy The surgical repair of a hernia.
kubaga umutsi nsoza bwenge	neurectomy Excision of a section of a nerve.
kubaga umwingo	thyroidectomy Surgical resection of all or part of the thyroid.
kubaga urukoba	graft A piece of tissue surgically transplanted.
kubaga ururimi	glossectomy Surgical resection of the whole or part of the tongue.
kubaga urusina	splenectomy Surgical excision of the spleen.
Kubaga utubuye two mu mafyifo	nephrolithotomy Surgical removal of a renal calculus.
Kubaga uturingoti two mugisusu	hemorrhoidectomy Surgical excision of a hemorrhoid.
kubaga uturingoti twumukoyo	ureterectomy Surgical resection of one or both ureters.
kubaga utuvyimba two mumubiri	enucleation Surgical removal of a globe.

Kirundi	English
kubagwa agasaho k'umusenyi k'urusogi	appendectomy Surgical excision of the appendix.
kubagwa mu gisusu	proctectomy Surgical excision of the rectum.
kubaho	viable Referring to a fetus that can survive childbirth.
kubangikana	adjacent, to be To be in proximity to.
kubira icuya	sweat, to The action of releasing moisture through pores of the skin.
kubira icuya	perspire heavily, to To sweat more than one would normally.
kubira icuya cane	diaphoretic Exhibited by profuse perspiration.
kubira icuya n'ijoro	night sweats Profuse sweating at night occurring with tuberculosis among other conditions.
kubira y'uwuringanizi	incoordination Absence of smooth, efficient body movement.
kuboga	vomit the mother's milk, to
kubogoza	sob, to To cry uncontrollably.
kubona ivyijiji	vision, blurred Haziness of the visual field.
kubonana na muganga	see the doctor, to
kubondoka	bloated Sensation of having an abnormally large amount of air in the viscera.
kuboneka	available Attainable, obtainable.
kubonerana	clear Transparent.
kubora kwigihimba cumubiri	necrosis The death of most of the cells of the affected part.
kubora kwuturingoti twamazi yo mumubiri	hidradenitis Inflammation of a sweat gland. When there is purulent discharge it is called hidradenitis suppurativa.
kubora umubiri (bivuye mukumara igihe kirekire uryamye)	decubitus ulcer A wound caused by laying in one position for too long; also referred to as a pressure ulcer.
Kuboregwa	dipsomania Compulsion to drink alcoholic beverages.
kuborerwa	alcoholism An addiction to alcohol.
kuborerwa	drunk,to be Inebriated.
kubura impemu	air hunger The sensation of shortness of breath.
kubura impemu	hypoxia Diminished oxygen content.
kubura impwemu	traumatic asphyxia Cyanotic asphyxia due to trauma. Extravasation of blood into the skin and conjunctivae caused by a sudden increase in venous pressure from a crush injury.
kubura inguvu	asthenia Diminished strength and energy.
kubura umukoyo	anuria The lack of urine excretion.
kubuyabuya	anxious Experiencing nervousness or unease.
kubuza	prevent, to To stave off or hinder.
kubwa	according to
kuchukwa mimba	gestation The development of a fetus from conception until birth.
kucyira icyungiro	disarticulation Amputation through the joint.

Kirundi	English
kudadarara umubiri	neurapraxia Paralysis from nerve injury but no degeneration of the nerve.
kudadarara umunwa	trismus Commonly called lockjaw, it is a spasm of the muscles supplied by the trigeminal nerve and is an early symptom of tetanus.
kudahwa amaraso	hematemesis Vomiting blood.
Kudahwa umwanya wose	cyclical vomiting Periods of recurrent vomiting with no apparent pathologic cause and the person has a normal state of health between the episodes.
kudashuha (eg.he is afebrile: Ntashushe)	afebrile Absence of fever.
kudatemebreza ibihimba vyumubiri neza	ataxia Lack of muscular coordination.
kudigadiga	tickle, to To lightly touch a person to cause one to laugh.
kudomako urutoke	localize,to Toward one point or area.
kudundura	bulge, to Formation of a protuberance on a flat surface.
Kufungura nabi	eating disorder General term for pathologic eating habits.
kugaba, gukanura	awakening The state of being conscious.
kugabanya	alleviate, to
kugaburirirwa mu mara	enteral feeding Nutrition supplied via the alimentary canal.
kugdegedwa	tremble from fear, to
kugena	ascertain, to Synonym of "to determine".
kugenda	ambulate, to Relating to walking.
kugenda	walk,to
kugenyera	circumcise, to To surgically excise the foreskin.
kugera	approximate, to To bring together, as in wound margins.
kugereka	add, to To count.
kugereza umurwayi mu gitanda	wash in bed Bed bath.
Kugigimiza	dysarthria Difficulty in articulation of speech.
kugigimiza	stammer,to The impulse to repeat the first letter of words and involuntary pauses while speaking.
kugigimiza	stutter,to Involuntary repetition of the first consonant.
kugira ibiro	overweight To be above the normal body mass index (BMI).
kugira amagura n amaboko bitangana	anisomelia Unequal size of arms or legs.
Kugira amaraso mugikiriza	hemothorax The abnormal presence of blood in the pleural cavity.
kugira amazi make mugitereko, kumugore yibungenze	oligohydramnios Inadequate amount of amniotic fluid.
kugira ibirenge bibase	flatfoot (to have) Common term for pes planus.
kugira ifuro ku munwa	froth at the mouth, to To have a mass of saliva with small bubbles in it coming out of the mouth.
kugira intege	weak,to be Feeble or deconditioned.
kugira intoke nke	oligodactyly Presence of fewer than 5 digits on a hand or foot.
kugira isangaya ryo mumutwe	concussion Head trauma resulting in temporary loss of consciousness.
kugira mikorobe nyinshi mu maraso	sepsis A condition exhibited by overwhelming inflammation due to infection.

159

Kirundi	English
kugira umushatsi muke	oligotrophia or hypotrichosis Less than normal amount of head/body hair.
kugirwa inama; imyimenyerezo	physical therapy Treatment of disease by heat, massage and exercise as opposed to medications.
kugisusu	perineal Referring to the perineum.
kugomorera	assistance The act of helping.
kugotwa	hypersensitivity Abnormal increase in sensitivity.
kugumbaha (1)	sterile 1. Infertile 2. Refers to equipment that is free of contamination.
kugumya	sustain, to To keep or maintain.
kuha	endow, to To supply or provide for.
kuhamagara	mention, to Refer to or allude to.
kuhenesha idzjicho	ectropion Eversion of the eyelid, usually the lower lid.
kuhindura amatariki	postpone, to To delay.
kuhinika	steatopyga Excessive accumulation of fat in the buttocks.
kuhunyayara	sprain, to have a A joint injury without fracture.
kuhurutura; kukorar'inda	labor, pre-term Onset of labor prior to the expected date of birth.
kuja mu kwezi	menstruation, to have
kuja mubutinyanka	ovulation The release of an ova from the ovary.
kuja mukwegi umwigeme akabura urubuto rusohoka	anovulatory cycle A menstrual cycle in which no ovum is released.
kuja mukwezi gake	oligomenorrhea Infrequent menstruation or low volume menstrual flow.
kujijura (gutuma imbanyi ivuka ningoga)	induce, to Facilitated. When referring to labor, it means medication was given to assist in delivery of the fetus. (induce labor)
kujujuta	abnormal, to be
kukomera	injury, to have an To have a wound.
kukwega itabi	snuff Chewing tobacco.
kumanuka	descending Moving toward the inferior portion.
kumata	adherence To stick to something figuratively or literally.
kumena inda	eviscerate,to The removal of bowels from the body.
kumeneka umutwe uruhande rumwe	cluster headache A unilateral, severe, recurrent headache.
kumenya	acquaint, to To make someone familiar with something.
Kumenya abantu nibintu	gnosia Ability to recognize things and people.
kumenyekana	known,to be Recognized or familiar.
kumerereza	goose bumps Cutis anserina.
kumira	deglutition The process of swallowing.
kumira	swallow, to To cause something to pass down the esophagus.
kumotera	olfactory Referring to the sense of smell.
kumugara	paralyzed, to be To not be able to move one or more extremities.
kumugara igice c umubiri	diplegia The paralysis of both arms or both legs.
kumugara igice co mumaso bivuye kukutetera kw umutsi nsoza bwenge ugira indwi	Bell's palsy Unilateral facial paralysis related to dysfunction of the seventh cranial nerve.

Kirundi	English
kumugaza	atrophy of a paralyzed extremity
kumva ingoma mumatwi	tinnitus Medical term for ringing in the ears. It is associated with Meniere's syndrome among other conditions.
kunamba	weight, to lose
kunamba cane	cachexia Generalized weakness and severe wasting.
kuniga	choke To retch, cough or fight for breath.
kuniga	gag,to To choke or retch.
kuniha	sigh,to A long deep exhalation that expresses an emotion, as in relief.
kunonosora ivyirwa vyo kubaga	orthopedics A surgical specialty concerned with treatment of skeletal problems.
kunuka	stink,to To have a foul odor.
kunuma	quiet,to be Making little or no noise.
kununuza	suck, to As in, to suction fluid.
kunya	defecate To discharge feces from the rectum.
kunyara	micturate,to Synonym of to urinate.
kunyaragura	polyuria Abnormal increase in volume of urine excreted.
kunyinyura	smile, to To spread the mouth with the edges upright.
kunyoganyoga	waddling gait Walking in short steps in a swaying fashion.
kunyunyuka	emaciated,to be To be abnormally thin and weak.
kunywa	drink, to To imbibe.
kunywa itabi	smoke, to To inhale on a cigarette.
kuraba	faint,to To lose consciousness.
kuragar'ingovi; ingovyi	placenta The vascular tissue that nourishes a fetus through an umbilical cord.
Kuragura	sorcery Black magic or voodoo.
Kuramba	long-standing Having existed for a long time.
kure	away from Separated from.
kurenga	beyond, to go To go further.
kurenza iariki yokuvuka	post-term birth An infant born after the normal length of pregnancy.
kurenza urugero rwumuti	overdose An above normal dose of a medication.
kuribwa mumushishito	retching Spasm of the stomach without presence of gastric material.
kurira	weep, to To shed tears.
kurokoka	recover,to (from a serious ailment)
kuromora	addiction An abnormal dependency.
kuronka imiti	medicine, to get
kuruha	tired,to be Fatigued.
kuruhuka mugitanda bisabwe na muganga	bed rest A medical order requiring one to stay in bed.
kuruhukira cane mugitanda	restless, to be Wriggle or squirm. Extreme restlessness, tossing around in bed.
kuruka	emesis,to have an To vomit.
kuruka	vomit,to The gastric contents that are expelled through the mouth.
kurumika	blood-letting The removal of blood from a patient with the thought it would cure or prevent disease.

161

Kirundi	English
kururirwa	bitter (taste) Having a harsh, unpleasant taste.
kururumba	febrile, to be To have a fever.
kurwara izosi	torticollis A condition exhibited by the head being turned to one side continuously.
kurwazwa n ubumara bwicunyunyu cam Plomb	lead poisoning The ingestion of lead, exhibited in severe cases by paralysis, encephalopathy, purple gingiva, and colic.
kurya	eat, to To consume food.
kurya canke kunywa	ingestion The intake of food or liquid orally.
Kurya-Guhekenya inzara zo ku ntoke	onychophagia Habitually chewing on one's fingernails.
Kuryama ugaramye	decubitus Laying flat in bed or dorsal decubitus. (lateral decubitus is flat and on one's side)
kuryamira umugongo ucuramye	trendelenburg position Position in bed in which the head is lower than the feet.
kuryarisha	labor onset The time when a pregnant woman begins uterine contractions in the process of childbirth.
kusarara	aphonia The loss of voice.
Kusokora	extubation The removal of a tube that was in a body orifice.
kutafungura	aphagia The lack of eating.
kutagend\a neza kitarico	negative Contrary or opposing.
kutagira amavya	anorchous The absence of testicles.
kutagira ubwenge bukwiye	amentia The absence of mental ability.
kutahembera	anosmia Lack of the sense of smell.
kutamenya	loss of consciousness Unresponsive to verbal and tactile stimuli.
kutamenya gusoma	alexia Inability to read due to a central brain lesion.
kutanyeganyega	stasis Lack of movement.
kutapata usingizi; ukubura itiro	insomnia Sleeplessness.
Kutarinda	agoraphobia The fear of being in a large open space.
kutatanya	inevitable, to be Not preventable.
kutawona kure	myopia Nearsightedness.
kutayobora ukuboko	athetosis An involuntary symptom exhibited by continuous slow, writhing movements, mostly in the hands.
kutetemera igice cumubiri	hemiparesis Unilateral muscle weakness (half the body).
kutimba kwakamirampeke	palatoplegia Paralysis of the palate.
kututisha ururimi	slurring Indistinct yet comprehensible speech.
kuva amaraso	bleed, to Loss of blood.
kuva amaraso mu gitereko	uterine bleeding Bleeding that emanates from the uterus.
kuva amaraso mu gitereko	metrorrhagia Uterine bleeding in normal amounts but at irregular intervals.
kuva amaraso mu kanwa, indwara yibura rya vitamine c	scurvy A disease of vitamin C deficiency exhibited by bleeding gums.
kuva amashira	purulent Referring to pus.
kuva amashira	suppuration Formation of purulent material.
kuva amazi	weep, to To ooze fluid, such as from a wound.
kuva 'masozi	lacrimation The secretion of tears.
kuvimba ikitigo	hepatomegaly Enlargement of the liver.

162

Kirundi	English
kuvimba urwagashya	splenomegaly An abnormally enlarged spleen.
kuvoma amazi mugitereko	amniocentesis Transabdominal aspiration of amniotic fluid.
kuvoma amazi mumubiri yo kuja gupima	aspiration biopsy Removal of fluid from a cavity for pathologic analysis.
Kuvoma amazi munda	abdominocentesis Puncturing of the abdominal wall for drainage purposes.
kuvoma amazi munda	paracentesis A procedure involving aspiration of fluid from the abdominal cavity.
kuvra 'maraso	hemorrhage,to have a Bleeding from a damaged blood vessel.
kuvubga	bereaved, to be The sorrow one feels with the loss of a loved one.
kuvuga	speak,to To talk.
kuvuka	born, to be Being present as a result of birth.
Kuvuka atanguje amaso	face presentation Referring to the part of the body coming out of the cervix first during childbirth.
kuvuka umwana atanguje umutwe	brow presentation The term used to describe which part of the body (forehead) is being delivered first in childbirth.
kuvuna	break, to (as in bone) A common term for a fracture in a bone.
Kuvunagurika kwamagufa	fracture, comminuted A broken bone where one segment overrides the other.
kuvundira mu gitanda	bedridden Term used to indicate one is so ill they cannot get out of bed.
kuvungagurika	friable,to be Easily reduced to powder.
kuvungavunga	nursing care, to give The assessment and treatment provided by nurses.
kuvunika amagufa yo mu gikiriza	flail chest The term used when one has multiple rib fractures causing a segment of the chest wall to move incongruently with the rest of the chest wall.
kuvunika ku rutugu	dislocation, shoulder Separation of the humerus from the scapula at the glenohumeral joint.
kuvura	treat, to Medical care one receives for illness or injury.
kuvura indembe y indwara y umutima n amahaha	cardiopulmonary resuscitation Use of artificial means to support respiration and circulation.
kuvura kwamaraso	hemostasis The control of bleeding.
kuvurwa cane	intensive care Vigorous treatment of the acutely ill.
kuvuza imiti, canecane ku ndwara ya kanseri	chemotherapy Use of medication (chemical agents) in the treatment of disease. This term is commonly used to refer to the treatment of cancer patients with medication.
kuvyara	deliver,to (a child) The process of giving birth. (forceps delivery)
kuvyaza umwana yicaye	breech birth Delivery with the feet or buttocks coming first.
kuvyimba	swell, to
kuvyimba amaguru	ankle edema or dependent edema Extracellular fluid volume noted by swelling or pitting.
kuvyimba amaguru	nonpitting edema Subcutaneous swelling that cannot be indented with compression.
kuvyimba ijisho ryikirenge	ankle swelling Enlargement of the ankle region with or without pitting.

Kirundi	English
kuvyimba inda	swollen (distended) abdomen
kuvyimba kwumutsi utwara amaraso wo kwizosi	jugular venous distension Enlarged jugular veins caused by high pulmonary capillary pressure.
kuwara	sick, to be
kuwira wyuya	ooze, to To slowly leak.
kuwiza icyuya cane	hyperhidrosis Excessive perspiration.
kuyonga kwamaraso	hemolysis Breakdown of hemoglobin.
kuyunguruka	rotation Movement around an axis.
kuzana	bring, to To carry or transport something.
kuzana amashira	fester, to To become infected.
kuzererwa	dizziness,to have Sensation of losing one's balance.
kuzibira	occlusion A pathway that is blocked or obstructed.
kuzibirwa impweno	dyspnea Difficult breathing.
kuzib'inda	intestinal obstruction Blockage of the intestine by mass or volvulus.
kuzimangana	blurred vision Low visual acuity. (fuzzy vision)
kuzungagiza	agitate, to To cause a state of extreme emotional disturbance.
kuzura	exhumation To remove a dead body from a grave.
kwa tombora	at random Occurring by chance alone.
kwaduka	flare-up A sudden worsening one's condition.
kwambura	disrobe, to To remove clothing.
kwandukira	contagious, to be Description of a disease that can be spread by direct or indirect contact.
kwandukizu	infectious disease Any disease or condition considered contagious.
kwandurutsa	provoke, to To evoke or elicit.
kwasamura	sneeze, to To suddenly expel air from the nose and mouth because of nasal irritation. (a sneeze)
kwaturura	burst, to To rupture.
kwayura	somnolence Drowsiness.
kwayura	yawn,to Opening one's mouth and inhaling deeply due to sleepiness/boredom
kwemera	approve, to Accepting something as satisfactory.
kwera	deciduous teeth,to get one's first or The first teeth.
kwibaruka biciye mu bihimba vy'irondoka	vaginal birth Delivery of an infant through the vagina.
kwicara	sit, to
kwidedomba	mumble, to To speak quietly and indistinctly.
kwigizayo igihimba c umubiri	abduct To move a body part away from the body.
kwihagararako, 2. kurinda 3. kugira Ishaka (depends on the context)	stamina Ability to maintain physical or mental exertion for a long period.
kwihangana	bear, to To endure or resist.
kwihangana	patient, to be To be unhurried.
Kwiherezo	distal Situated away from the center of the body.
kwiherezo	peripheral Referring to an outward part or surface.
kwikunda cane	narcissism Abnormally excessive self-interest.

Kirundi	English
kwima	withhold, to To refuse to give something.
kwimenya	cope, to To deal with a difficult situation.
kwimyira	blow one's nose, to
kwinjiza umuntu mu bitaro	admission (to hospital) To be admitted.
kwinyugunura indobo	brush teeth, to Use of a toothbrush to clean the teeth.
kwinyugunyura	gargle, to To rinse one's mouth out and exhale through the liquid.
kwiraba (verb), imirabu (noun)	tattoo A design made by inserting indelible ink into the skin.
kwirabura umubiri bivuye mu kubura impwemu mu mubiri	cyanosis Bluish discoloration of the skin and mucous membranes.
kwirwaza	malinger,to To feign illness.
kwitfatisha ibipimo vyuzuye kwa muganga	physical exam Examination of a client to assess their medical status.
kwitonganya	whisper,to Speech in a volume that is barely discernible.
kwituma amaraso	melena The passage of black, tarry stools indicative of upper gastrointestinal bleeding.
kwituma amaraso yirabura	black stools Common term for melena.
kwiyagaza mumatwi	ringing in the ears Common term for tinnitus.
kwiyahaza	pruritus A general term for conditions exhibited by itching.
kwiyawira icyubu	desquamation The shedding of scales of any body surface.
kwiyitumako	encopresis Involuntary defecation.
kwiyugara	stenosis Narrowing of an orifice.
kwizana	spontaneous Occurring without provocation.
kwizera	reliable Trustworthy.
kwoma	comply, to Adhere to.
kwonda	thin Lean or slender.
kwondesha	thin, to become To lose a lot of weight.
kwongereza amazi	hydrate,to To replenish fluid balance.
kwongeza	accelerate (To accelerate the healing process).
kwonka	suckle, to An infant taking to his mother's nipple.
kwonka; kwonsa	nurse, to To suckle or feed a baby at the breast.
kwonsa	breast feeding The process of giving milk to a baby via the nipple.
kworoha	soft,to be Easy to mold or compress.
kwoza igisabo	douche Cleansing of a canal; unless otherwise specified it refers to cleansing of the vaginal canal.
kwubika inda	prone Lying with the abdomen and face downward.
kwuma mumubiri	heat exhaustion A condition that occurs secondary to prolonged exposure to high ambient temperature; it is exhibited by subnormal temperature, dizziness and nausea.
kwumva	feel, to To perceive or discern.
kwumva bihurugushwi	hard of hearing,to be Decreased sense of hearing.
kwumva umuntu ariko arahema	breath sounds The noise heard upon auscultation with a stethoscope.
kwumva uwugukozeko	sensation A perception when one is touched.
kwumviriza	taste,to Sensation of flavor perceived in one's mouth.
kwunyuka	exacerbation Worsening of an existing problem.

165

Kirundi	English
kwunyuka	worsen, to To deteriorate.
kwuzur inda	dyspepsia Indigestion.
kwuzurana	saturation An amount, expressed in a percentage, that expresses the degree something is absorbed versus the maximal absorption possible.
magoremagabo	hermaphrodite A person possessing gonadal characteristics of both sexes.
mbere	former Prior.
mburugu	chancre The initial ulcer that is seen with primary syphilis.
mu bwonko	meningeal Referring to the dura mater, arachnoid and the pia mater.
mu gikiriza	mediastinum The thoracic area between the lungs.
mu gisusu	anal Near or referring to the anus.
mu kirenge	plantar Referring to the bottom of the foot.
mu magage	oropharynx The portion of the pharynx between the soft palate and the superior aspect of the epiglottis.
mu migwi	serial In a series.
mu ntabarimbabare	emergency room A ward used for initial treatment of critical patients.
mubwonko	intracerebral Within the cerebrum.
mubworo bwikirenge	sole of foot Common term for plantar aspect of the foot.
muganga gorora abamugaye; abavunitse canke abahinyagaye	physical therapist Clinician who specializes in rehabilitation of persons with lower extremity disorders.
muganga ujejwe ingorane zo	psychologist Clinician with a doctorate degree who specializes in treatment of mental disorders without the use of medications.
muganga w'amaso	optometrist A person who practices optometry.
muganga w'amaso (muganga ubaga)	ophthalmologist A physician specializing in diseases of the eye.
muganga w'amatwi	audiologist A clinician specializing in disorders of the ear.
muganga w'ibirenge	podiatrist Physician, surgeon specializes in disorders of the feet.
mugiga	meningitis Inflammation of the meninges exhibited by fever, photophobia, nuchal rigidity and in severe cases coma and convulsions.
mugiga yo mumutwe	encephalitis Inflammation of the brain.
Mugiga yo mumutwe no mugiti cumugongo	encephalomyelitis Inflammation of the brain and spinal cord.
mugisusu	rectal Referring to the rectum.
muhure (ibicurane vyo mu muri wa B)	influenza Viral infection causing fever, muscle aches and catarrh. (hemophilus influenza B)
mukanwa	oral Relating to the mouth.
mukanwa	orally By mouth. (verbally)
mumagufa	intraosseous Within a bone.
mumazuru n imihogo	nasopharyngeal Referring to the nose and pharynx.
mumazuru n imihogo	nasopharynx The part of the pharynx which lies superior to the soft palate.
munini uzana amaras mu'mutwe	carotid Referring to the large artery on each side of the neck.

Kirundi	English
munsi	under; infra Sometimes used when indicating a patient is "under treatment" for a condition (active treatment).
munsi yimisaya	submaxillary Situated below the maxilla.
munsi yururimi	sublingual Situated under the tongue.
munsi yurwara	subungual Under a fingernail or toenail.
muntege	popliteal fossa The hollow in the posterior aspect of the knee joint.
murukoba	transdermal Through the skin.
mutoya	young Having lived for a short period.
muzitsa	wisdom tooth Third molar.
mw'ivyariro	maternity Area of the hospital where women deliver babies.
neza	positive Indicating the presence of something.
nico gituma	hence Thus.
nka	approximately Nearly but not completely.
nk'ibise	contractions Abdominal muscle contractions during the last weeks of pregnancy.
nuko; niko	right Sure, agreed, OK (adverb)
nyamuragi	aphasia Diminished ability to communicate via speech or writing.
nyamwero	albino A person who lacks pigment in the eyes, skin and hair.
nyayo	specific Clearly defined.
n'indwara bukumbi y'ubwonko	cerebrovascular accident (stroke) A decrease in level of consciousness and paralysis caused by a cerebrovascular thrombosis, hemorrhage or vasospasm.
n'indwara bukumbi y'ubwonko	stroke Common term for cerebrovascular accident.
n'ubwo	despite Notwithstanding.
n'urushinge batera mu ruti rw'umugongo	epidural anesthesia Injection of medication in the epidural space for pain control. Commonly used during childbirth.
pia ya mguu; iyitfu m'ivi	kneecap Common term for patella.
pia ya mguu; iyitfu m'ivi	patella The bone situated in the anterior portion of the knee.
prostate (ari ko gasabo gakikije umuyoboro usohora inkari ku mugabo).	prostate A gland found in men that surrounds the neck of the urethra and bladder.
radial> igihande co hejuru yukoboko	radial Referring to the radius.
rimatizime	rheumatism Any condition exhibited by inflammation and pain in the joints and muscles.
rimwe mumagufa agize ikiyunguyungu	ischium The inferoposterior portion of the pelvis.
rugagamisha	microscope A instrument used to magnify and view small objects.
rwose	absolutely
serumu	serum The fluid that isolates out when blood coagulates.
sida	Acquired Immunodeficiency Syndrome (AIDS) Presence of an AIDS defining illness or having a CD4 of less than 200/mm3.
SIDA	AIDS Acquired Immunodeficiency Syndrome

Kirundi	English
sutama; indwara y umwanda	typhoid fever A condition caused by ingestion of food or water containing salmonella typhi that is exhibited by fever and abdominal signs and symptoms.
tetanosi	tetanus A condition caused by Clostridium tetani which produces spasm and rigidity of voluntary muscles.
tifoyide	mite fever Synonym of typhus fever.
tinfusi	typhus fever A rickettsiae infection exhibited by rash, fever, headache and myalgia.
ubgana	childhood The time between infancy and puberty.
ubgiba	confinement As in confined to bed.
ubgonko; ubwonko	brain A common term for cerebrum.
ubgoya {inzia}	hair (of body) {axillary and pubic hair}
ububabare	discomfort A feeling of physical or mental unease.
ububabare	pain Physical suffering or discomfort.
ububabare igihe ubutinyanka	dysmenorrhea Pain during menstruation.
ububoneke	appearance The way someone looks or presents.
ubucafu	dirty Unclean.
ubucuti	empathy To be concerned for and share the feelings of another.
ubugari	width Side to side measurement.
ubugaru	talipes equinovaro Medical term for what is commonly known as club foot.
ubugugu	debility Physical weakness.
ubuhanga bw'ukuvura abatama	geriatrics The study of the health of old people.
ubuhanza	alopecia The absence of hair in areas where it normally exists.
ubuharura	scrape An injury caused by having a body part rubbed against a rough surface.
ubuhinga bwo guhemera mu matwi	Valsalva's maneuver A technique in which one attempts to exhale with the mouth and nose closed; this equalizes pressure in the ears.
ubuhinga bwo kubaga	marsupialization Creation of a surgical pouch.
ubuhinga bwo kufata amaraso mu mitsi	phlebotomy The removal of blood for testing or as a therpeutic intervention.
ubuhinga bw'ukwiyumvira n'inyifato	psychology The study of the human mind and emotions.
ubukangwe	poliomyelitis An infectious viral disease exhibited by constitutional symptoms that can lead to quadriplegia.
ubukene	deficiency Insufficiency or deficit.
ubukene	need A want or obligation.
ubukongatare	paraplegia Paralysis of the lower extremities.
ubukuru	age Length of life.(old age)
ubukurugutwi	cerumen Waxy substance found normally in the external ear canals.
ubukurugutwi	wax Cerumen.
ubukwe	marriage The formal union of a man and a woman.
ubumara	toxin A poison of plant or animal origin.
ubumara	venom (snake) A term used to describe the toxin injected via a bite or sting.

Kirundi	English
ubumenyi	cognition The process of acquiring thought or understanding.
ubumenyo buhanitse	learning The intentional acquisition of knowledge.
ubumote	odor A smell that is given off someone or something.
ubumuga	deformity A malformation or imperfection.
ubumuga	disability Decreased or impaired mental or physical ability.
ubumuga	impairment A specific disability.
ubumuga	weakness Feebleness.
ubumuga bwamagufa yo mumisaya	micrognathia Abnormally small maxilla or mandible.
ubumuga bw'ubuvukano	birth defect A congenital anomaly.
ubunini	size The dimensions of something.
ubupfamatwi	deafness Having impaired hearing.
ubupfunya	atrophy A diminution in the size of a part.
uburake; ishavu	anger A strong feeling of annoyance or hostility.
uburambe	longevity Long life.
uburebure	height Distance between the bottom of the foot and top of the head.
uburebure	length The end to end measurement.
ubureme	density The denseness of an object.
ubureve	defect, speech A shortcoming or imperfection in speech.
ubureve	lisping A speech problem in which "s" and "z" are pronounced "th".
uburiba	weight
uburibwe	ache A mild pain
uburire	conjunctivitis Inflammation of the conjunctiva.
uburire	pink eye Common term for acute contagious conjunctivitis.
uburiri	bed A mattress resting on a frame.
uburozi	poison A substance that causes illness or death.
uburuhe	fatigue Tiredness and exhaustion.
uburuhukiro	morgue A room where deceased patients are housed until sent to a funeral home.
ubururu	blue A color between green and violet.
uburyo	right When referring to the right hand or side.
uburyo ataco bushikanako	ineffective Unsuccessful or inefficient.
uburyo bwo kuvyara kurugero	contraceptive A device or medication used to prevent pregnancy.
ubusasate	itch A sensation that makes one want to scratch.
ubusaza	old age A relative term for the period of advanced years.
ubusazi	Alzheimer's disease A dementia of unknown cause or pathogenesis.
ubusazi	dementia A chronic brain disorder exhibited by memory loss, personality changes and faulty reasoning.
ubusazi	insanity Referring to a serious mental illness.
ubushe	burn An injury caused by exposure to heat.
ubushe buvuye kubukanye	frostbite Local tissue destruction after exposure to cold.

Kirundi	English
ubushe bwimitsi itwara amaraso	arteritis Inflammation of an artery.
ubushobozi bwo kwumva inkintu ugikozeko	stereognosis The ability to identify an object by touch.
ubushuhe	heat The quality of being hot.
ubushuhe	temperature The degree of internal heat in a person's body.
ubushuhe buza bukagenda	undulant fever Wave-like variations in the fever, going from very high to normal and back again, as seen in Brucellosis.
ubushuri	triplets Three infants born during one birth.
ubusinziriza	trypanosomiasis A disease caused by a protozoa of the genus Trypanosoma that can cause sleeping sickness and Chagas' disease.
ubusunwa bw'urutoke	fingertip Distal aspect of a finger.
ubutinyanka	amenorrhea The absence of menses.
ubutinyanka	menses The blood and other material expelled from the uterus during menstruation.
ubutinyanka	menstruation Synonym of menses.
ubutinyanka bubabaza	menstrual cramps
ubutinyanka cane	menorrhagia Abnormally large amount of menstrual blood.
ubutinyanka y'icambere	menarche The time of the initial menstrual period.
ubutumbi	distension Swollen.
ubuvyibuhe	corpulence Fatness.
ubuvyimbe	inflammation Localized redness, excessive warmth and swelling.
ubuvyimbe bw'isaho nkingiramara	peritonitis Inflammation of the peritoneum.
ubuyabaga	adolescence
ubuyoya	infancy Early childhood.
ubuzima bwose	lifetime Duration of a person's life.
ubwami bwikirenge bunini	pes cavus Excessive height of the longitudinal arch of the foot.
ubwicariro	gluteal or gluteus muscle A paired set of three muscles, the gluteus maximus, medius and minimus, that all have origins in the ilium and insertions in the femur. (buttocks)
ubwinjiriro bw'igitereko	cervix uteri The narrow end of the uterus.
ubwinshi	plethora An excess of something.
ubwiyahuzi	suicide To kill oneself intentionally.
ubwoba	phobia An profound fear of something.
ubwoko bw abasirikare b umubiri	neutrophil A polymorphonuclear leukocyte.
ubwoko bw imibango	knock knees Common term for genu valgum.
ubwoko bw Imirazi	exotropia A type of strabismus that is characterized by the eyes turned outward.
ubwoko bw umutsi	muscle, latissimus dorsi
ubwoko bw umutsi	muscle, oblique

Kirundi	English
ubwoko bw umutsi wo kwitako	muscle, quadriceps
ubwoko bw umutsi wo mugikiriza	muscle, pectoral
ubwoko bw umutsi wo mumugongo	muscle, trapezius
ubwoko bwabasoda bumubiri	basophil A polymorphonuclear granulocyte.
Ubwoko bwabasoda bumubiri	monocyte A leukocyte with an oval nucleus and grey cytoplasm.
Ubwoko bwabasoda bumubiri bita Eosinophil	eosinophil A cell with eosin stain used to designate a type of leukocyte that is elevated during allergic reactions.
ubwoko bwinkabuyo	fibrin An insoluble protein formed when fibrinogen is acted upon by thrombin.
ubwoko bwumusonga	sharp (pain) When describing pain, a piercing sensation.
ubwoko kw inkabuzo	keratin A protein found in the skin, hair, nails and enamel of the teeth.
ubwome	glue Plastic cements
ubwonko n uruti rw umugongo	central nervous system (CNS) The brain and spinal cord.
uduce twamahaha	bronchiole A small branch that a bronchus divides into.
udukore sho babohesha uwavunitse	brace A splint.
udutemere two mu mitsi itwara amaraso	aortic valve The valve situated between the left ventricle and the aorta.
udutsi nsanganya maraso	capillary A vessel that connects arterioles to venules.
uguca imvyaro	menopause The time when menstruation ceases.
ugucandaga	vaccination The act of receiving a vaccine.
ugufata	laxity A description of a joint that is loose.
ugufuta	cool Chilly or cold.
uguhagarara umutima	congestive heart failure A diminished cardiac output leading to passive engorgement.
uguhanga	gaze Steady, intent look.
uguhembera	lactation The secretion of milk from mammary glands.
uguhezera	wheeze
uguhushanya	contradication A situation in which two elements are inconsistent.
uguhuza	matching Corresponding in pattern or style.
uguhuza ibitsina	coitus Sexual intercourse between members of the opposite sex.
ugukakaza vitari 'vigirankana	involuntary movement Movement not controlled consciously.
ugukama amazi	dehydration The status of having a decrease in total body water.
ugukina kwumwana	fetal movements Sensations by the mother of fetal activity.
ugukira	healing The process of becoming healthy again.

171

Kirundi	English
ugukora ku	contact The touching of two bodies or a person who has been exposed to a contagious disease.
ugukora nabi kw' inkingiramubiri	immunodeficiency An inadequate immune response.
ugukumira	quarantine A place of isolation for infectious persons until it can be certain it is safe to let them mingle.
ugukura	growth The increase in physical size.
ugukura	resection The removal of tissue.
ugupfa kw ubwonko	brain death Cessation of cerebral functioning.
ugupfa kwinyama yumubiri kubera iura ry amaraso	ischemia Inadequate blood supply to a part of the body.
Ugupima umuti	dosing interval The number of times per unit a medication is given.
ugupima urugero rwinzoga mu maraso	blood alcohol level A quantitative measurement of the amount of alcohol in the blood.
ugusarara	hoarse A rough, harsh sounding voice.
ugushika	access Means of entry.
ugushima kw'umwigisha	comment A remark providing an opinion.
ugushoboka	likelihood The probability or feasibility.
ugusiramura	circumcision The surgical excision of foreskin.
ugusohora impwemu	breathing
ugusohora umurwayi mu bitaro	discharge,hospital The release of a patient from the hospital.
ugusokora	withdrawal The action of being without drugs or alcohol.
ugusuka intanga	ejaculation The emission of semen at the moment of sexual climax in a male.
ugusuzuma umuvyimba	autopsy Examination of a body post-mortem in an attempt to determine cause of death.
ugusuzuma umuvyimba	necropsy Synonym of autopsy.
uguta umutwe	disorientation Mental confusion.
ugutakaza akayabagu	anorexia The loss of appetite.
ugutandukanya imvyaro	family planning Birth control.
ugutanga	distribution The manner in which something is shared or spread out.
ugutanga akayaga	ventilation The movement of air into the lungs; generally meant to suggest by an artificial process.
ugutanga umuti	dosage The amount and frequency a medication is given.
ugutenga	bandage A strip of gauze used to immobilize or support.
ugutimba kwingohe	ptosis Drooping of the upper eyelid usually due to paralysis of the third cranial nerve.
ugutimba nk'igiti	paresis Incomplete paralysis.
ugutobora	perforation Presence of a hole.
ugutunganya	management The process of dealing with things or people.
ugutura ingiga	drowsiness Sleepiness.
ugutwi	auricle The external portion of the ear.
ugutwi	ear The organ of hearing and balance.
Ugutwi kwimbere	ear, inner Auris interna.
Ugutwi kwinyuma	ear, middle Auris media.

Kirundi	English
ujejwe ingorane zijanye no	speech therapist A person trained to assist people with speech and language disorders.
ujejwe kunonora imitsi ku kazi	occupational therapist A clinician who specializes in rehabilitation of persons with upper extremity disorders.
ujejwe kuraba ko abantu bafungura neza	dietician Clinician specializing in the treatment of nutrition related disorders.
uko umuntu aboneka	external Outside of the body.
ukubaga (kubaga)	operation A surgical procedure. (to operate)
ukubamfu	hand, left
ukubara	evaluation Assessment or evaluation.
ukubenja kwamaso y abana	jaundice of the newborn A form of jaundice seen in newborns in the first two weeks of life; also called icterus neonatorum.
ukuboko (amaboko)	arm One of two upper extremities. (arms)
ukuboko canke ukuguru	extremity Refers to one arm or one leg.
ukuboko kw'ibubamfu	arm, left
ukuboko kw'iburyo	arm, right
ukubona	vision State of being able to see.
ukubona (kubiri)	diplopia Double vision.
ukubona ibiri kure guza	hyperopia Farsightedness.
ukuboneka	availability A person or thing that is available.
ukuboneka	emergence Coming into prominence.
ukubora kw'amenyo	caries Referring to decay or death of a tooth.
ukuborewa	inebriation Intoxication with drugs or alcohol.
ukububika amazi munsi y'urukoba	edema Extravascular fluid accumulation.
ukubura ihemero	suffocation To die from a lack of air or inability to breathe.
ukubura impwemu	asphyxia A condition exhibited by a lack of oxygen and subsequent loss of consciousness or death.
ukubura ingaburo	malnutrition Lack of appropriate nutrition.
ukudadarara kw'imitsi	convulsions An involuntary series of tonic and clonic movements.
ukudakora kw'igihimba c'umubiri	failure, organ The cessation of function of body organs.
ukudedemda (kudedemba)	delirium;to be delirious An acute mental state exhibited by altered thought processes and restlessness.
ukudihagizwa (kudidagira)	palpitation Sensation of a forceful, rapid, irregular heartbeat present after exercise or with anxiety.(to have palpitations)
ukugabanya	analgesia The absence of pain.
ukugobeka	insertion The act of inserting something.
ukugumbiza	fecal impaction The presence of hard excrement in the rectum that requires manual removal.
ukuguru	leg One of two lower extremities.
ukugwiza amakopi	duplication The process of duplicating something.
ukujana	compliance The act of going along with a plan.
ukundi	again Once more.
ukunuka mu kanwa	halitosis Foul odor emanating from the mouth.

173

Kirundi	English
ukunyinganga uradahwa	motion sickness Nausea associated with travel.
ukuraba	blackout Common term for loss of consciousness.
ukuraba	coma A state of unconsciousness.
ukuraba	faint Weak and dizzy.
ukuraba	stupor A reduced level of consciousness.
ukuribwa mu matwi	earache Pain associated with the ear.
ukurondoka kw'abantu	fertility The ability of a person to contribute to contraception.
ukuruhira ubusa	abortion (miscarriage) Premature expulsion of the fetus from the uterus.
ukuruhira ubusa	miscarriage Spontaneous abortion.
ukurwazwa n'indya zityoye	food poisoning Poisoning where the active agent is in the food.
ukutakira inkomezi mpuzabitsina	impotence Inability to act or inability to achieve a penile erection.
ukuva amashira (igituba)	discharge, abnormal vaginal Purulent vaginal secretions.
ukuva amashira (ugutwi)	discharge, ear Otic secretions.
ukuvyara ku rugero	birth control Any method of limiting contraception.
ukuvyimba imiriro	pharyngitis Inflammation of the pharynx.
ukuvyimba imiriro	sore throat Common term for pharyngitis.
ukuvyimba kwamahaha	high altitude pulmonary edema
ukuvyimba kwubwonko	high altitude cerebral edema
ukuvytara	parturition The process of giving birth.
ukuwuku/ukuguru	member Referring to an extremity (arm or leg).
ukuzinduka uradahwa	morning sickness Nausea associated with pregnancy.
ukuzitira utaronerwa	prophylaxis That which is done to prevent disease.
ukwagura	enlargement Becoming bigger.
ukwagura	expansion Enlargement or increase in size.
ukwaha	armpit A common term for axilla.
ukwaha; ubwakwaka	axilla The hollow beneath the arm.
ukwibuka	recollection Memory.
ukwica	homicide When one person kills another.
ukwima	deprivation The lack of a necessity.
ukwinjiza impwemu	breathing in
ukwinjiza impwemu	inspiration Drawing in a breath.
ukwirukana	expulsion Evacuation or elimination.
ukwisobako	incontinence Inability to control urination.
ukwitera umwino	enema A procedure involving insertion of fluid into the rectum.
ukworoherwa	relief Alleviation from pain or discomfort.
ukwumva	hearing Auditory perception.
umegera w amagufa n imitsi	osteomyelitis Inflammation of the bone or bone marrow because of a microorganism.
umonga w'ukuwoko	antecubital fossa The hollow at the bend of the elbow.
umti winkorora	antitussive Medication used to diminish a cough.
umubabaro	morbidity The state of disease.
umubiri	body The physical structure of a person.

Kirundi	English
umubiri uboze	**infarct** Referring to dead tissue.
umubiri usaneza	**asepsis** Lack of infection.
umubiri uvyimvye	**induration** An area that is abnormally hard.
umubiri wavyimvye	**puffiness** Having a soft, swollen area.
Umubiri woboze	**cuticle** The dead skin at the base of the toenail or fingernail, also called the eponychium.
umuco	**light** Illumination, bright.
umudzi	**nerve** A fibrous band made up of axons and dendrites that connects the nervous systems with other organs.
umudzi w'amaraso urarimvye	**aneurysm** A condition exhibited by the dilatation of the walls of an artery or vein to form a blood-filled sac.
umudzi w'amatwi	**auricular nerve** Nerve supplying the ear.
umuforomo (umuforomokazi)	**nurse** A person trained to care for the sick.(female nurse)
umufyiri	**black** Referring to the color, as in the color of coal.
umugabo	**man** Male human.
umugaga (utusaduke ku'ikiworo)	**fissure** A general term for a cleft or deep groove. An anal fissure, for example, is a small ulcer adjacent to the anus. (anal fissure)
umuganga	**physician** Medical practitioner.
umuganga abaga	**surgeon** A physician who performs surgery.
umuganga bw'indwara zo mu mutwe	**psychiatrist** A doctor who treats persons with problems of the human mind and emotions and can prescribe medication.
umuganga wa kanseri	**oncologist** A physician specializing in the treatment of cancer.
umuganga w'abana	**pediatrician** Physician who is a specialist in pediatrics.
umuganga w'amenyo	**dentist** A professional capable of treating diseases of the teeth and gums.
umugera	**bacteria** Plural for any organism of the order Eubacteriales.
umugera	**sting** A small puncture as in a bee sting.
umugera w indwara y urukoma	**anthrax** An infectious disease caused by Bacillus anthracis; there are cutaneous, inhalation and gastrointestinal syndromes.
umugera w urukoba	**herpes** A skin condition exhibited by formation of clustered vesicular lesions; herpes simplex is at times referred to, albeit incompletely, as herpes.
umugera wa herpes	**shingles** A reactivation of herpes zoster.
umugera wa SIDA	**HIV** Abbreviation for human immunodeficiency virus.
umugera wa virus y urukoba	**herpes zoster; shingles** A unilateral vesicular rash along one dermatome and caused by inflammation of a posterior nerve root by "the chicken pox virus".
*umugera wo ku gashino *(names of genital parts sound impolite, better to say . Umugera wo mubihimba vyirondoka)*	**wart on clitoris**
umugera wo mukirenge	**plantar wart** A viral epidermal growth on the bottom of the foot.
umugera wubushuhe uterwa nimibu (umupfube)	**yellow fever** A viral, hemorrhagic fever transmitted by mosquitos.

175

Kirundi	English
umugera w'indwara	germ Microorganism.
umugimbi	child A person aged 1 to 8 years old. (male, female)
umugiraneza	volunteer A person who performs work without expecting compensation.
umugoma	blood clot A mass of coagulated blood.
umugombero	tibia The larger of two long bones in the lower leg.
umugongo	back The back of a person.
umugongo (kurwara)	back pain Discomfort on the dorsal surface of the torso.
umugore ataratwara inda	nulligravida A woman who has never been pregnant.
umugore ataravyara	nullipara A woman who has never given birth.
umugore yibungenze	pregnant woman
umugororo	clavicle A bone that articulates with the sternum and scapula.
umugororo	collarbone Common term for the clavicle.
umugwayi	patient The client being treated for a medical or surgical condition.
umuhinga mu n'imiti	pharmacist A professional who prepares and sells medicine through various systems, including governmental organizations like the Veterans Administration.
umuhiro y'amatako	skin fold An overlapping of skin formed by subcutaneous tissue.
umuhogo	pharynx The membranous cavity from the mouth to esophagus. (umio is sometimes used to describe esophagus at also the larynx)
umuhogo	throat The anterior aspect of the neck.
umuhondo	colostrum The fluid secreted by the mammary glands a few days around parturition.
umuhondo	yellow A color between green and orange in the spectrum
umuhurudutsi	rude Ill-mannered.
Umujigiti; uburoso bwo koza amenyo	toothbrush Handheld instrument used to clean one's teeth.
Umukasi wo gushona	needle holder A surgical instrument used to grasp a needle during suturing.
umukasi wo kubaga	scissors A cutting instrument with two blades, joined at the middle.
umukenke w'ukumuwiriz' awarwaye	acoustic Referring to the auditory system.
umukerecu	strain, knee Knee pain severe enough to prevent one from walking.
umukoba	labia majora The folds of skin forming the lateral borders of the pudendal cleft.
umukobga	daughter
umukondo	navel Umbilicus.
umukondo	umbilicus The scar that denotes the end of the umbilical cord.
umukoyo urimwo isukari	glycosuria Presence of glucose in the urine.
umukoyo urimwo proteini	proteinuria The presence of protein in the urine.
umukuba	current Flow or stream.

176

Kirundi	English
umukunzi	magnet A piece of iron with atoms ordered to make it magnetic.
umukwabu	scratch A long, narrow superficial wound.
umuntu agendana umugera wa SIDA	AIDS, person living with
umuntu akuze	adult Generally considered a person over 18 years old.
umuntu w'inkone	eunuch A man who has been castrated.
umunuko	odiferous Having an unpleasant or distinctive smell.
umunwa	labium Referring to any lip shaped structure.
umunwa	lip The fleshy tissue surrounding the mouth.
umunwa mubi	cleft lip A congenital abnormal opening of the lip.
umunwa wo hasi	lip, lower Labium inferius oris.
umunwa wo hejuru	lip, upper Labium superius oris.
umunya	sodium chloride A colorless, crystalline compound; also table salt.
umunyu	saline A solution of sodium chloride.
umunyu	salt Typically referring to sodium chloride.
umunzane	scale A device to check a person's weight.
umunzane upima inzoya	baby-scale A device used to weigh an infant.
umurabu wumuhondo uva kwigwirirana ryibinure kurukoba	xanthoma A lipid deposition on the skin exhibited by an irregular yellow patch.
umuramu	abrasion Superficial skin injury.
umurazi	cataract An opacity of an eye lens or the capsule.
umureberebe	leech An annelid used in some tropical regions for drawing out blood; they have an anticoagulant effect locally and have been attached to digits of persons with acute peripheral ischemia.
umurenda	mucous A substance secreted by mucous membranes.
umurindi w'amaraso	blood pressure Written as the measurement in mmHg at the time of systole of the left ventricle over the time of diastole.
umuringoti binjiza mumubiri wo kwa muganga	indwelling catheter Continuous use tube usually referring to a tube in the urinary bladder.
umuringoti utwara amaraso wo munda	aorta The large artery originating at the left ventricle and going to the pelvis where it bifurcates.
umurinoti wo gushira mumushishito	nasogastric tube A tube that is inserted into the nose with the distal tip in the stomach; it is used for irrigation or drainage of gastric contents.
umuriro	pyrexia Fever.
umuriro; inyonko	febrile Presence of an supraphysiologic temperature.
umuriro; ubushuhe	hyperpyrexia Fever.
umuriro; ubushuhe	hyperthermia Fever.
umurongo ngenderwako	scheme A program or plan.
umurongoro	rectum The terminal portion of the digestive tract extending from the distal sigmoid to the anus.
umuruga	scrotum The sac which contains the testes.
umurundi	fibula The smaller of two bones in the lower leg.
umurundi	shin Refers to the anterior tibial region.

177

Kirundi	English
umurungoro	colon The portion of the large intestine that goes from the cecum to the rectum.
umurwayi	pediculosis Lice infestation.
umurwayi	sick person
umurwaza	caregiver A person who provides care to another.
umurwi wamaraso	blood grouping Testing blood to determine which type should be used for transfusion.
umurwi w'amaraso	blood type Determined and listed in the ABO system.
umurya	tendon Fibrous tissue that connects muscle to bone.
umurya w'umugongo	vertebral column The cervical, thoracic and lumbar vertebrae.
umusangwabutaka	indigenous Naturally occurring.
umusanzi w'inzu	nap A brief sleep or catnap.
umusarani uvanze n amavuta	steatorrhea Excrement with an abnormally high fat content.
umusarani, amazi avanze nibirenduka	stool, watery with mucous
umusarani;amavyi	excrement Feces.
umusaya	temple The temporal fossa superior to the zygomatic arch.
umusaza	elderly Advanced in years.
umusegetera	mosquito net A fine mesh fabric hung over a bed as a mosquito repellent.
umusego	cushion A pillow or stuffed pad used to sit on.
umusego	pillow An encased fabric covering soft material used for a cushion.
umusemoro	insect bite
umushatsi {ubwanwa}	hair (of head) {facial hair- beard}
umushikanuro; ikifube	epileptic seizure A convulsion related to abnormal brain activity (as opposed to being precipitated by hypoglycemia.)
umushiro	disappearance An instance of something/someone gone missing.
umushitsi (kuja mu gashitsi)	shiver A trembling. (to shiver)
umusikati	nasal bone
umusimbi	mons pubis The prominence over the symphysis pubis in a female caused by a fat pad.
umusino	labia minora The folds of skin enclosed in the pudendal cleft within the labia majora.
umusoda womu mubiri	antibody A protein that combines with and counteracts foreign substances.
umusokoro	bone marrow The soft material filling the cavity of bones.
umusonga	pneumonia Inflammation of the lung due to an infection caused by a virus or bacterium.
umusonga muryinyo	ocular paralysis. Paralysis of intraocular and extraocular muscles.
umusonga mw ibere	mastodynia Breast pain.
umusonga ufata imitsi yo mumaso	tic Periodic spasmodic facial muscle contractions.
umusonga ushinga nkicumu	stabbing pain A sharp piercing quality to pain.
umusonga waho baciye igihimba	phantom limb pain Pain sensed in an area where one has had an amputation as though the limb is still present.

Kirundi	English
Umusonga wo kururimi	glossodynia Tongue pain.
umusonga wo mu matwi	otalgia Ear pain.
umusonga wo munda	guarding A symptom used to describe a patient resisting an examination because of severe pain; often seen in patients with peritonitis.
umusonga wo mw ivya	orchialgia Testicular pain.
umusoso	hip The lateral eminence of the pelvis from the waist to the thigh; it is formed by the iliac crest and greater trochanter.
umusumbi	hypogastrium The area of the central abdomen located below the stomach.
umusumeno	saw A hand or power-driven tool used for cutting.
umusyegenyo	friction Grating or rasping.
umutari	bright Giving out a lot of light.
umuti	cure A remedy for a medical illness.
umuti	elixir A medical solution.
umuti	tablet A small disk of a compressed solid substance.
umuti	medicine A substance used for medical treatment or the art and science of healing patients.
umuti ; uwuruzi	medication A substance used for medical treatment.
umuti mponyamigera	antibiotic A medication that inhibits or kills microorganisms.
umuti ugabanya ububabare	analgesic A medication used to remove pain.
umuti uhonya imigera	disinfectant A substance that kills bacteria.
Umuti Ukiza	curative A remedy capable of healing completely.
umuti ukora umwanya muremure	long-acting Referring to a drug with long lasting effects.
umuti uvura uburozi bwiyindi miti	antidote A medication that neutralizes a toxin.
umuti wanditswe n'umuganga	prescription The action of prescribing a medication or treatment.
umuti wibikomere	swab An absorbent material used for cleaning wounds or applying ointment.
Umuti winyongera	adjuvant Term used to describe the medical treatment after initial therapy, as in adjuvant radiation therapy after initial chemotherapy.
umuti winyonko	antimalarial Medication used to treat malaria.
umuti wo guhwamika	tranquilizer A medication used to diminish anxiety.
umuti wo gutimbisha	anesthetic A chemical that produces anesthesia.
umuti wo kudahwa	antiemetic A medication used to control nausea.
umuti wo kunywa	syrup A thick sweet liquid.
umuti wo kwica intanga	spermicide A substance capable of killing sperm.
umuti wubububabare	opium An addictive drug derived from opium poppy; synthetic versions are used as analgesics.
umuti wubumara bwinzoka	antivenin An antitoxin formulated for various types of snake bites.
umuti wuduhere two kurukoba	antipruritic Medication used to treat pruritus.
umuti wumutwe	antimigraine Medication used to treat headaches.
umuti w'amenyo	toothpaste

179

Kirundi	English
umuti; ikinini	pill A medicated tablet or capsule.
umutima	heart Muscular organ that pumps blood thru the circulatory system.
umutima n imitsi yamaraso	cardiovascular Referring to the heart or circulatory system.
umutima uratera vuba	high blood pressure Elevated arterial blood pressure.
umutima uratera vuba	hypertension Higher than normal blood pressure.
umutima utera buhoro	hypotension Abnormally low blood pressure.
umutima utera bukebuke	bradycardia Lower than normal cardiac rate measured in beats per minute.
umutsi	blood stream (blood vessel) Common term or the arterial or venous systems.
umutsi utwara amaraso wo kwizosi	jugular vein (s) Includes the internal, external and anterior jugular veins.
umutsi uvana amaraso mu mutima	artery Vessel that carries oxygenated blood from the heart to the periphery.
umutsi wo kurutugu	muscle, deltoid
Umutsi womukuguru	gastrocnemius A large muscle in the lower leg, responsible for ankle plantar flexion, that is attached to the distal femur and achilles tendon.
umutwe	caput The head.
umutwe	head
umutwe w'imboro; intini	glans penis The distal aspect of the penis.
umutwe w'uruhande rumwe	migraine An episodic, unilateral headache accompanied by nausea.
umuvukanyi	sibling A brother or sister. (younger sibling)
umuvurngano	confusion Disorientation.
umuvyazi	midwife A person trained to assist in childbirth.
umuvyeyi afise imvyaro nyinshi	multipara A woman with more than one live births.
umuvyeyi amaze kwibungenga kenshi	multigravida A woman who has been pregnant more than once.
umuvyimba	cadaver A dead body.
umuwango	rickets A condition exhibited by softening and bowing of the long bones; caused by Vitamin D deficiency.
umuwanzo	onset The beginning of an event.
umuyaya	heat stroke A condition caused by excessive exposure to high ambient temperature; it is exhibited by dry skin, thirst, vertigo, muscle cramps and nausea. The three forms are heat exhaustion, heat cramps and sunstroke.
umuzi wiryinyo	pulp The tissue filling the root canals of a tooth.
umuzimbwe	anal ulcer An open wound near the anus.
umwaka	year A time period that covers 365 days.
umwambiro	yeast A unicellular fungus.
umwana (abana)	baby A newborn.(babies)
umwana ahema nabi	fetal distress Term used to describe an abnormal heart rate or rhythm in a fetus indicating the need for urgent childbirth.
umwana akiri munda	embryo The term used to describe a fertilized ovum in the first 8 weeks of development.
umwana arafuye mu'nda	stillborn Refers to a newborn that died in utero.

Kirundi	English
umwana yicaye	breech presentation Position of the feet or buttocks near the cervix.
umwanda mukuru wa mberew umwana	meconium The first newborn feces which are green.
umwanda muto;inkari; amasobe	urine The fluid concentrated by the kidneys and expelled via the urethra.
umwanya	interval An intervening time.
umwararo	perineum The area between the anus and scrotum or anus and vulva.
umwenge	meatus, urethral Orifice at the entrance of the urethra.
umwenge y'izuru; itondi	nostril One of two openings in the nose used for air passage.
umwete	application The forms one fills out to obtain a grant.
umwidodombo	complaint Grievance.
umwikanzi	nightmare An unpleasant or frightening dream.
umwingo	goiter Swelling of the thyroid gland.
umwinizirano	cecum The first portion of the large intestine.
umwiriri	nose, bridge of
umwiriri	nose, tip of the Distal aspect of the nose.
umwuhagiro	bathing To wash oneself.
umwuka wubumara	carbon monoxide poisoning This tasteless, odorless gas causes constitutional symptoms but can lead to death upon inhalation.
umwuka, impwemu	oxygen A colorless, odorless gas with atomic number 8.
umwuna	epistaxis Bleeding emanating from the nose.
umwuna; ikicyurane	nosebleed Common term for epistaxis.
unyongonyo	malaise A vague feeling of discomfort or unease.
uracuye ku'mugongo	prolapse of the rectum Terminal portion of the rectum comes through the anus.
urubavu	rib One of a series of curved paired boney articulations protecting the thorax.
urubibe	demarcation Having a fixed boundary.
uruboyi	bee sting A piercing from a bee.
urubu	clot A thrombus or embolus.
urubu	sour An acid or bitter taste.
urucanco	vaccine A solution of attenuated microorganisms given to prevent or treat a disease.
urucandago	immunization A medication given to provide immunity.
urucange	compound A substance formed by covalent union of two or more atoms.
urugenda rw'imirindi	intermittent Occurring at irregular intervals.
urugero	amount The total or the aggregate.
urugero	flow Movement in a continuous stream.
urugero	rhythm The pattern or cadence.
urugero	span A distance between two objects.
urugero rwo hejuru	high Elevated.
urugero umutima utererako	heart rate Number or cardiac contractions per minute.
urugohe (ingohe)	eyelash Each of the short hairs on the eyelid.(eyelashes)
uruguma	cut An incision.

Kirundi	English
uruguma rwo kumutwe	head trauma Any injury to the brain.
uruhago	bladder, urinary Vestibule for urine prior to being expelled via the urethra.
uruhago	urethra The canal connecting the urinary bladder with the outside of the body.
uruhago	urinary bladder The organ collecting urine from the ureters prior to discharge via the urethra.
uruhanga	forehead Section of the face from the hairline to the eyebrows.
uruhekenyero; amagage	palate The roof of the mouth.
uruhere	eruption of pustules Initial onset of a cluster of pustules.
uruhongore rw'ingurube	sty Also called hordeolum externum, it is inflammation of the sebaceous gland of an eyelash.
uruhorihori	fontanelle or fontanel The space between the bones in the skull that are separate at birth.
uruhu	dermis The "true skin" that lies beneath the epidermis.
urukebu	stiff neck Not easy to bend the neck without referring to a cause.
urukenyerero	pelvis The boney structure connecting the spine with the legs.
urukenyerero	waist The part of the body between the ribs and the hips.
urukoba	epidermis The skin cells overlying the dermis.
urukoba rwo kumushatsi	scalp The skin covering the head except for the face.
urukoba rwonze	pachydermia An abnormally thick skin.
urukoba rw'umutwe w'imvyarabibondo	foreskin Also called prepuce, the skin that naturally covers the glans but can be rolled back.
urukonda	polysialia Abnormal increase in saliva.
urukumu	thumb The first digit of each hand.
urukushi	urticaria A diffuse pruritic macular rash, caused by an allergy.
urumogi	marijuana Cannabis.
urunyuzi	suture Thread used for sewing together a wound.
urupfu	death The action of dying.
ururabwe	glance A brief look at something.
ururasago	cicatrix (scar) New tissue in a healed wound.
ururasago	incision An intentional surgical cut in the skin.
ururenduka	mucous plug A mass of mucous and cells that forms in the cervical canal during pregnancy.
ururimi	tongue The fleshy muscular organ of the mouth.
urusagusagu; urusakanwa	chin Mentum; the anterior projection of the lower jaw.
urusato; umuhiro	skin Flesh.
urushi w'ukuwoko	scapula Medical term for the shoulder blade.
urushinge	needle The slender cylindrical device attached to a syringe.
urushinge	syringe A device used for administering medication through various routes.
urushinge rwa parasitike rwo gucishamwo umuti	catheter A flexible tube inserted into the body.

Kirundi	English
urushinge rwo gupimisha	needle biopsy Use of a needle to aspirate body contents for microscopic or pathologic examination.
urusina	ascites Serous fluid in the abdominal cavity.
urusina	cirrhosis A liver disease characterized by destruction of liver cells and increased connective tissue.
urusoro; imbuto	fetus Medical term for the infant prior to birth.
uruti rwumugongo	supine Flat on one's back.
uruti rw'umugongo	spine The spinal column or a thorny protrusion.
urutirigongo	backbone Spine.
urutoke	digit Finger.
urutoke	finger Any of the five digits on the hand.
urutsure	glare An angry stare.
urutuga	shoulder The joint were the scapula joins the clavicle and humerus. (right shoulder, left shoulder)
uruvya	prostatitis Inflammation of the prostate gland.
uruvyaro	offspring One's children. (child)
uruvyaro rwambere	primipara A woman giving birth for the first time.
uruwe	sleeping sickness Also called Trypanosomiasis, this disease is caused by a parasitic protozoa and transmitted by the tsetse fly.
uruyoya; umwana mutoyi	neonate The term for a newborn infant for the first four weeks.
uruyoya; uruhinja	infant Newborn.
uruzingo	sick child
uruziri	leukorrhea Thick white vaginal discharge.
uruziruzi	amniotic fluid The fluid surrounding the fetus.
uruzogi	umbilical cord The stalk between the placenta and the unborn infant.
urwakashaya	spleen The visceral organ that is involved with production and removal of blood cells.
urwambariro	ankle joint The articulation of the tibia/fibula and talus.
urwara	fingernail Thin horny plate over the dorsal aspect of the end of finger.
urwara	nail The hard surface on the dorsal surface of the toes or fingers.
urwara	toenail The nail at the tip/dorsal aspect of each toe.
urwego rwumuntu. Ingaragu vs uwubatse	marital status Single versus married status.
urwibagiza	anomia Inability to name or recognize familiar objects.
urwoba	fungus A spore-producing organism that feeds on organic matter.
urwubati	sheath A covering.
ususarani	feces Excrement.
utuhere	vesicle A blister.
utuherehere	chalazion A chronic inflammatory granuloma of a meibomian gland; also called meibomian cyst.
utuherehere	meibomian cyst An enclosed fluid collection along a sebaceous gland of the eyelid.

183

Kirundi	English
uturingoti imbuto zicamwo	oviduct The channel which an ovum passes from the ovary.
uturingoti twimbuto	fallopian tubes Either of a pair of long narrow ducts located in a female's abdominal cavity that transport the male sperm cells to the egg.
utwininga	regardless of Without consideration of.
uwagize	casualty A person who is killed or seriously injured.
uwara w'amata	jejunum The portion of the small intestine from the end of the duodenum to the ileum.
uwegendakanwa	glossitis Inflammation of the tongue.
uworoshi; kinyoganyoga	flaccid Limp. A term applied to an extremity one cannot move actively.
uwugegeni	amputation Typically referring to the surgical removal of a limb.
uwuhemyi	inhalation The act of breathing in.
uwuhinduzi	inversion Turning inward.
uwuhomyi	gauze A fabric used for dressing changes.
uwuhuguto.	infection A contagious disease.
uwukarabe	crust Dried serous exudate covering a wound.
uwukumbutsi	memory Ability to remember.
uwura w'amata	intestine, large Portion of the bowel from the ileocecal valve to the rectum.
uwura w'amayoge	intestine, small The portion of the small bowel extending from the pylorus to the ileocecal valve.
uwuremere	inertia The tendency to remain unchanged.
uwuriri	layer A stratum or thickness.
uwuronderezi	on going Continuing,
uwurozi	toothless Edentulous.
uwuryi, inzara nyinshi	bulimia Chronic condition characterized by secretive eating of large quantities of food followed by self-induced vomiting.
uwusazi	hysteria A psychological condition exhibited by uncontrolled emotion or exaggerated manifestations.
uwusazi	madness Common term for insanity.
uwusazi; uwuzeze	mania A mental disorder exhibited by hyperexcitability, delusions and euphoria.
uwutukure	jaundice Yellowing of the sclerae and skin because of excessive bilirubin in the blood.
uwuwawazi w'ikiwuno; ikinyamukinya	low back pain Pain in the lumbar region.
uwuwawazi w'ikiwuno; ikinyamukinya	lumbago Pain in the region of the lumbar spine.
virahongodotse	tooth, chipped A tooth with a small piece broken off.
vyihuta	urgency Emergency or priority.
vyinshi	lots of An abundance of.
Vyuka	get up out of bed
w'ijoro	nocturnal Referring to events that happen at night.
w'urwinubwe rurenze urugero.	paranoia To have delusional thoughts.
y'imbere	internal Situated on the inside.
y'imisumbi	inguinal Referring to the groin.

184

Kirundi	English
y'inyuma; amongero	accessory Complimentary or concomitant.
y'ukurisha	nutrition The process of supplying food needed for growth.
y'umutima	cardiac Referring to the heart.
zero	zero No quantity.

Other books by A.H. Zemback

English-Kinyarwanda-French Dictionary

English-Kinyarwanda Dictionary

English-Kirundi-French Dictionary

English-Kirundi Dictionary

English-Swahili-French Dictionary

English-Swahili Dictionary

English-French Medical Dictionary and Phrasebook

English-Spanish Medical Dictionary and Phrasebook

English-German Medical Dictionary and Phrasebook

English-Portuguese Medical Dictionary and Phrasebook

English-Italian Medical Dictionary and Phrasebook

Medical Kinyarwanda Phrasebook and Glossary

Medical Swahili Phrasebook and Glossary